# The HeartMath Solution

# The HeartMath® Solution

Doc Childre and

Howard Martin,

with Donna Beech

HarperOne
*An Imprint of HarperCollinsPublishers*

HarperOne

FIRST HARPERCOLLINS PAPERBACK EDITION PUBLISHED IN 2000

*Library of Congress Cataloging-in-Publication Data*
Childre, Doc Lew
    The HearthMath solution : the Institute of HeartMath's revolutionary program for engaging the power of the heart's intelligence / Doc Childre and Howard Martin with Donna Beech. —1st ed.
        p. cm.
    ISBN: 978–0–06–251606–0
    1. Psychophysiology. 2. Heart. 3. Emotions. 4. Emotions and cognition. 5. Brain.
I. Martin, Howard. II. Beech, Donna. III. Institute of HeartMath. IV. Title.
QP360.C48    1999
613—dc21                                                                98–55300

09 10 11 12 RRD(H) 30 29 28 27 26

## Dedication

This book is dedicated to facilitating the millions of people who are wanting to learn more about aligning the mind with the heart and to those who are realizing that it's time for practical emotional management skills to survive and thrive in today's changing world.

## Important Note for the Reader

The material in this book is intended to provide an overview of the new research related to the role of the heart in well-being. This research is extensively referenced for readers wishing to pursue further inquiries and study. Every effort has been made to provide the most accurate, dependable, and current information. Any suggestions for techniques, treatments, or lifestyle changes referred to or implied in this book should be undertaken only with the guidance of a licensed physician, therapist, or healthcare practitioner. The ideas, suggestions, and techniques in this book should not be used in place of sound medical therapies and recommendations.

# Contents

# Part 4: Social Heart Intelligence   225

# Foreword

It's rare that one comes across a solution that goes well beyond the original problem, yet that's been the case for me with the evolving work of HeartMath.

In modern life we hear references to the heart in many different contexts: we feel love in our "heart" or we feel a "heart connection"; we give our "heart" to a project or our work; we take a compliment or criticism "to heart"; our courage is a measure of our "heart"; we "come from the heart" when we act with compassion. Yet what does "heart" really mean in these everyday expressions? Certainly the word doesn't refer to the organ called the heart that I studied during medical training—an organ that pumps each and every second to supply the oxygen and nutrients within the blood to our cells throughout the body.

Western conventional medicine speaks of the heart solely in terms of its physiological function. In that medical definition, the heart is a multichambered muscular organ crisscrossed with electrical circuitry. The heart is often described as a pump and the arteries as pipes—essentially the biological equivalent of the well pump and plumbing in your house. This description is in such marked contrast to our emotional sense of the heart that one is left wondering if there's any connection whatsoever between the literal and figurative, the physical and the mystical. This question underlies the HeartMath Solution, and its answer can have a significant effect on one's health and overall well-being.

The difference between the physical and emotional definitions of "heart" is rooted in the body/mind split so pervasive in medicine today. We've separated the role of our thoughts and daily stresses from the effects that they produce in the physical body. Throughout their medical training, physicians are told of bacterial, metabolic, toxic, and other causes of physical illness, yet the relationship of our thoughts and emotions to effecting physical change is for the most part ignored. This has in large measure led to a medical model that can be dehumanizing, focusing solely on the specific physical manifestations of disease, thus losing sight of the whole person.

The response among concerned healthcare professionals to this body/mind split has been the development of fields such as psychosomatic and behavioral medicine and, more recently, studies in psychoneuroimmunology. To heal this split, new practices have evolved that have been termed "holistic" or "complementary" or "integrative" — practices that seek to integrate and address the full spectrum of body, mind, and spirit. HeartMath — whose beauty lies in its simplicity and profundity — is one such approach.

As a physician, I've become fascinated by the relationship between time and health. Most of us in modern society feel that we never have enough time — a feeling that results in the frenzy and hurry that underlie all our stress and lead to serious diseases and disorders. Recognizing that time is the rhythmic dimension of life, I've begun to see that health is a delicate balance of rhythm, while dis-ease results from dis-rhythm. In a time where chaos and disrhythm are part of everyday life, it's essential that we develop exercises that help reestablish and regulate normal rhythms and thus promote health. The work that Doc Childre and Howard Martin present here in *The HeartMath Solution* shows a significant way to change patterns and rhythms within the physical body, restoring health through understanding the heart as more than just a physical pump and seeing how the rhythms themselves are regulated by love.

This book shows in depth, how the heart is at the core of our body and at the core of how we think and feel. The "solution" is derived from realizing that the heart is both a physical object, a rhythmic organ, and love itself. It recognizes the heart as the central rhythmic force in the body and shows us how to use the coherent power of love to manage our thoughts and emotions. Like a pebble that creates a ripple of waves when dropped into a still pond, so love and positive feelings in the heart create a rhythm that spreads health and well-being throughout the body. In modern medicine this is difficult to understand, because of our tendency to separate and differentiate mind and matter, emotions and the physical body, instead of recognizing the interconnection between them.

When I first came across HeartMath, I was struck by the unusual combination of scientific research and emotional wisdom. I was familiar with studies suggesting that meditation or thinking good thoughts can make a person feel better, less depressed, or healthier, but these studies could be considered "soft" science. Here, though, were studies showing significant changes in patterns of heart rate and blood chemistry. HeartMath represents an important point of convergence: truly showing the impact of feeling love, compassion, and gratitude on underlying physiological conditions. This work clearly demonstrates that using the exercises of HeartMath can profoundly affect our health and have a positive effect on the way we think, feel, work together, and relate in all aspects of life.

If we take this book seriously, we'll forever look at ourselves, others, and the world around us very differently. HeartMath research confirms our intuitive understanding of the heart with solid science and explains how the electromagnetic field radiating from the heart can affect those around us. HeartMath tools and techniques show us how to move from linear thinking to intuitive sensing, providing greater intelligence and creative solutions to our present and future challenges.

The HeartMath Solution holds promise for a society that sees science as its religion and requires scientific studies and results with significant numerical changes before credibility for the approach can be granted. The power of HeartMath is that it's rooted both in scientific research and understanding and in the wisdom of love. It gives a new—yet old—meaning to "heart" that embraces all aspects of what we know it to be.

*Stephan Rechtschaffen, M.D.*
*author of* Time Shifting *and president of the Omega Institute*

# Acknowledgments

The creation of *The HeartMath Solution* has been quite an experience from inception to completion. Although there are other books about specific aspects of HeartMath, this book was written in order to bring many of these elements together into one source while at the same time presenting new information, applications, and experiences gained over the last several years. In order to accomplish that goal and create a definitive book about HeartMath, we required the aid and support of many people.

Many friends and colleagues have spent years of dedicated service, both personally and professionally, developing and implementing the HeartMath system. Some of these people made valuable contributions to this book, and they'll undoubtedly continue to contribute in many ways (seen and unseen) to its success. We'd like to extend our thanks to them.

Many thanks to:

Sara Paddison, the president of the Institute of HeartMath, for her unwavering dedication, guidance, and direction and for her invaluable help on *The HeartMath Solution* project.

Deborah Rozman, the executive vice president of HeartMath LLC, for her immeasurable help in the writing of this book and for her contributions to the externalization of HeartMath through her background in psychology and her business skills, leadership, and public representation.

Rollin McCraty, director of research for the Institute of HeartMath, and his colleagues, for conducting leading-edge scientific research that is creating a new model of how we view the heart while improving the health of thousands of people.

Bruce Cryer, vice president of global business development for HeartMath LLC, and his team, who have taken this work so skillfully and effectively into corporations and organizations around the world.

Joseph Sundram, for his dedicated service in taking HeartMath into government agencies and the military, as well as to the disadvantaged, who need help so badly.

Jeff Goelitz and Stephanie Herzog, for the innovative contributions they're making in education and child development.

David McArthur, for his deep commitment to providing HeartMath to religious organizations of all kinds.

Jerry Kaiser and Robert Massy, for the groundbreaking work they're doing with healthcare providers and individuals with health challenges.

Special thanks to Kathryn McArthur, Dana Tomasino, Wendy Rickert, and Mike Atkinson for taking care of the many details required to complete this book.

There are many more people to appreciate, to say the least, so we thank you all for your sincere work, support, and deep friendship:

Much love and respect to all of the staff at the Institute of HeartMath, HeartMath LLC, and our partners and associates around the world.

We'd also like to thank the entire staff at Harper San Francisco for their belief in and support of *The HeartMath Solution*. Thanks also to Donna Beech, the fine collaborative writer who helped us throughout the writing of this book while making it even more fun, and to our agent, Andrew Blauner, who would definitely be a finalist for "The Most Sincere Literary Agent" award if it were ever given.

The hard work and sincere care that these many people have invested in this book are much appreciated.

*Doc Childre and Howard Martin*

# Introduction

The HeartMath system, from which *The HeartMath Solution* was derived, was created by Doc Childre, a stress researcher, author, and consultant to leaders in business, science, and medicine. HeartMath offers an innovative view of psychology, physiology, and human potential that provides a new model for efficient living in the modern world.

Doc has spent most of his adult life researching and developing the HeartMath system. His goal with that system has been to give people the ability to unfold new intelligence and more caring, compassionate feelings to help them meet life's many challenges with resiliency and poise. It was out of this sincere desire to help people that, in 1991, Doc, along with a small group of professionals representing a wide spectrum of talents, experience, and expertise, founded the Institute of HeartMath, a nonprofit research and educational organization. The Institute's research has made pioneering inroads into the fields of neuroscience, cardiology, psychology, physiology, biochemistry, bioelectricity, and physics. In order to further its research objectives, the Institute formed a scientific advisory board composed of leaders in many of the above fields to provide guidance and peer review. This collaboration has led to the exciting new discoveries that are presented throughout this book.

The HeartMath system's scientifically validated techniques have been integrated into seminars and consulting endeavors delivered by HeartMath LLC, the master training organization licensed by the Institute and headed by Doc Childre, and through their licensed trainers around the world.

Today the HeartMath system is officially being taught on four continents in a variety of societal contexts, including corporations, government agencies, healthcare institutions, and educational systems.

I've been a part of HeartMath's development for almost thirty years, playing many roles during the system's various stages of growth. During the last eight years, I've been primarily a businessman and HeartMath trainer/spokesperson.

Currently, I'm executive vice president, chief creativity officer, of HeartMath LLC, a sales marketing company that creates and publishes products based on the HeartMath system. These roles have placed me in a position central to much of what HeartMath is doing in the world. I've been given the opportunity to contribute to this book and express some of what I've learned about the heart, myself, people, and life during these many years. I'm honored to do so and sincerely appreciate the opportunity.

I began my discovery of the heart when I was a young rock musician living in North Carolina. As I was trying to make some coherent meaning out of a life that could only be characterized as quite chaotic, I started to listen to the voice of my heart. I found it often provided a reliable compass for making important decisions. That was motivation enough to keep going for more. Fortunately, my association with Doc and his work during this time offered me the chance to learn more. Developing a respect for the intelligence of the heart at a young age has been, by far, the most important contributor to my success in life.

One intention of this book is to confirm to you, the reader, what you may already feel or know—that the heart is involved in understanding yourself, people, and life. If you take to heart what you read and make even a small but sincere effort to apply what you learn, you'll experience a profound shift in your perceptions and emotions. Life will respond accordingly. It won't take years to benefit from the HeartMath Solution. In fact, it will save years of looking for answers that are only as far away as the shift from mind to heart.

Today, there's not enough time for everyone to take a leisurely approach to becoming more intelligent, caring human beings. Our current and future challenges require the discovery of new inner resources needed to change at a faster pace. The simple system offered in *The HeartMath Solution* shows you how to make a direct connection with the intuitive intelligence resource of the heart. As people develop this intelligence, it gives them the power they need to manage their mind and emotions and achieve a greater capacity to create positive changes in society.

*The HeartMath Solution* presents three types of information: concepts, tools and techniques, and biomedical, psychological, and social science research. The combination of these elements provides a comprehensive system for unlocking innate potential and achieving rapid personal, interpersonal, and social advancement.

In today's world many people put their faith in science and technology, gaining valuable knowledge, inspiration, and comfort from the breakthroughs and enhancements to living that science provides. Others intuitively sense that faith in science can be limiting, that something more is needed for fulfillment of the human spirit.

One of the exciting aspects of life at the cusp of the new century is that people are sensing the possibility of a merger between science and spirit. As you'll see in this book, our years of experience, practice, and research tell us that the heart is the doorway to this union.

Through the Institute's research, in conjunction with the research of others, we've been able to build a compelling case that the heart does have an intelligence that influences our perceptions. Our research challenge has been to see whether (and how) the philosophical or metaphorical "heart" and the physical heart interact. We've found that they indeed do, and in a number of ways. As impressive as much of what we've discovered is, however, there's much more to learn. Because available scientific instruments can't measure all the effects of the heart, the total picture isn't yet complete. Neurocardiologists and other scientists are just beginning to map the pathways and understand the mechanics of how the heart communicates with the brain.

Moving beyond what we've been able to prove through science, our theory is that the heart links us to a higher intelligence through an intuitive domain where spirit and humanness merge. This intuitive domain is something much larger than the perceptual capability of the human race has yet been able to grasp. But we can develop that perceptual capacity as we learn to do what sages and philosophers have asked us to do for ages: listen to and follow the wisdom of the heart.

We can learn a great deal from science, but we don't have to wait for science to prove *everything* before we can access the wisdom and intelligence of our hearts. Many people intuitively sense that such access is possible; in fact, they long for it—they just don't know how to achieve it. A reliable method is what they've been waiting for.

*The HeartMath Solution* offers a step-by-step methodology for people to develop the intuitive intelligence of their own hearts. It's not the only system for balancing the mind and emotions and contacting the heart's intuition, but it's one system that *works*. HeartMath is being successfully implemented by many thousands of people who systematically use the tools and techniques we offer to increase their awareness.

With stress increasing in the world, people are looking for ways to find more mental and emotional balance in their lives. As people wake up to new possibilities, they become motivated to better manage themselves mentally and emotionally in areas they've avoided or not known how to address. These people become the pioneers who lay the groundwork for others.

My hope in sharing this work is to help people experience a much larger degree of mental and emotional well-being, expanded awareness, and heightened fulfillment. One thing I've learned from practicing the HeartMath system is that fulfillment starts on the inside and then becomes evident on the outside where it can be appreciated the most.

If fulfillment that exceeds expectation can happen for me, it can happen for you. I sincerely believe that all of the good things that have come my way have done so because I learned how to listen to and follow my heart. *The HeartMath Solution* presents a way to do exactly that. On behalf of Doc and myself, *enjoy!*

*Howard Martin*

# PART 1

# Heart Intelligence

The HeartMath Solution is a comprehensive system that provides information, tools, and techniques to access your heart intelligence. Part I is designed to give you the foundation needed to take the first step of the HeartMath Solution: acknowledging your heart intelligence.

This first section will describe heart intelligence, explain how it works, and discuss why it's so important. Scientific research will be presented that reveals an intelligence residing within the heart and shows how the heart communicates with the brain and the rest of the body. This research has shown that when heart intelligence is engaged, it can lower blood pressure, improve nervous system and hormonal balance, and facilitate brain function.

In order for the mind, emotions, and body to perform at their best, the heart and brain must be in harmony with one another. Learning to align these two integrated but separate sources of intelligence is another important part of this section.

In Part I you will:

➢ Realize the significance of heart intelligence

➢ Understand the biological communication between the heart, the brain, and the rest of the body

➢ Distinguish the difference between the head and the heart

# CHAPTER 1

# Beyond the Brain—
# The Intelligent Heart

It was 5:45 A.M. on Tuesday morning, February 6, 1995. We were at Heart-Math's business center in Boulder Creek, California. Dr. Donna Willis, the medical editor for NBC's *Today* show, had called the previous afternoon to say that they'd decided to run a segment on our work the next morning. They were going to call it "Love and Health." Dr. Willis would start off with an overview of the Institute of HeartMath's research about the electrical energy produced by the heart. Then she'd go on to tell Bryant Gumbel and the viewers about our FREEZE-FRAME technique, which uses the power of the heart to manage the mind and emotions.

"We'll have only a few seconds to give them your number," Dr. Willis said, "but you might want to put some of your people on the phones, just in case."

With little time to prepare, we quickly arranged for our staff to come in early to handle any calls—and it was lucky we did! As soon as the phone number appeared on the screen, the switchboard lit up. For the rest of that day and into the night, then all day long the next day, we fielded calls almost continuously. Each time the show aired in a new time zone, another wave of calls came in.

We talked to thousands of people from all over the country—from anonymous parents in big-city ghettos to leaders in science, medicine, business, education, and religion. Before it was over, we'd gotten calls from around the world—all from a four-minute segment on a national television show that flashed our phone number on the screen for five short seconds. Why was that brief mention of the heart so magnetic?

The people who called us knew instinctively that the heart played an important role in their overall well-being. "I knew it all along," they said, and now they were eager to find out more. They wanted to know how their thoughts and feelings could be used to improve their health—mentally, emotionally, and physically. Others—people who associated the heart with love—wondered what they could do to bring more "heart" into their lives.

This immediate response further confirmed our long-standing belief that people are ready to put the heart to work in their lives. Without knowing the specifics, they sense that loving, positive feelings are somehow related to health, and they do their best to encourage those feelings in their lives.

Most people would rather feel loving and appreciative than resentful and depressed. But often the world around us seems to be spinning out of control. Despite our best intentions, it's hard to maintain our emotional equilibrium when we're confronted every day—sometimes every hour—with stressful situations.

We've all been told, at one time or another, to follow our hearts. And it sounds like a great idea, in principle. But the problem is that actually following our hearts—and loving people, including ourselves—is much easier said than done. Where do we begin? People *talk* about following their hearts, but nobody shows us how to do it. What does following the heart really mean? And how do we love ourselves? Aside from love's being a nice sentiment, why should we love other people? We'll show you a practical, systematic approach to answering these questions for yourself and outline the enormous benefits you'll reap in doing so.

Over the past twenty years, scientists have discovered new information about the heart that makes us realize it's far more complex than we'd ever imagined. We now have scientific evidence that the heart sends us emotional and intuitive signals to help govern our lives. Instead of simply pumping blood, it directs and aligns many systems in the body so that they can function in harmony with one another. And although the heart is in constant communication with the brain, we now know that it makes many of its own decisions.

Because of this new evidence, we have to rethink our entire attitude toward "following our hearts." At the Institute of HeartMath (IHM), scientists have found that the heart is capable of giving us messages and helping us far more than anyone ever suspected. Throughout this book, we'll share the research that provides new evidence of the power of heart intelligence. And we'll show how that intelligence can have a measurable impact on our decision-making, our health problems, our productivity at work, our children's learning ability, our families, and the overall quality of our lives.

It's time to reexamine the heart. As a society, we need to take the concept of heart out of confinement in religion and philosophy and put it right in the "street," where it's needed most. The HeartMath Solution is a comprehensive system that will give you new information about heart intelligence; new tools, techniques, and exercises to access that intelligence; and instructions and examples regarding how and when to apply it to make your life better.

The biomedical, psychological, and social science research presented in this book provides the underpinnings of the HeartMath Solution. As you learn and apply this system, you'll rapidly gain new solutions to problems, new insights, and an expanded understanding of yourself, other people, society, and life itself.

The heart isn't mushy or sentimental. It's intelligent and powerful, and we believe that it holds the promise for the next level of human development and for the survival of our world.

As we enter the new millennium, our increasingly global society is faced with daunting challenges. The world's power structures are changing. Leaders are suffering from a lack of credibility. Technology is rapidly linking the world through satellite TV and the Internet, creating both opportunity and challenge. More nations are gaining nuclear capabilities. Threats of terrorism, global weather changes, and uncertainty prevail. Many important institutions and systems that we rely on for security and order are in disarray.

Largely because of all this change, stress is at an all-time high. As Albert Einstein said years ago, "The significant problems we face today cannot be solved at the same level of thinking we were at when we created them." Developing the capacity to deal with the challenge of living in a stressful, ever-changing world is now more important than ever. To live happily and healthily in all the turmoil that progress brings requires exploring new ideas.

Hundreds of years ago it was obvious to everyone that the earth was flat. That fact was clearly observable; the earth extended as far as one could see. When the means to travel further and take a better look became available, however, everything changed. In the fifteenth century, the explorations of Columbus and Magellan proved to the world what Copernicus had already calculated mathematically: despite appearances, the earth is round. Then Galileo verified Copernicus's theory that the earth revolves around the sun, not the other way around. In the span of a few decades, our world had been turned upside down.

In the realm of the heart, the Magellans have returned with news of strange new lands. They tell us, "Our old models were based on limited information." [1] New discoveries now reveal that within each of us there exists an organizing and central intelligence that can lift us beyond our problems and into a new experience of fulfillment even in the midst of chaos. It's a high-speed, intuitive source of wisdom and clear perception, an intelligence that embraces and fosters both mental and emotional intelligence. We call it "heart intelligence."

Heart intelligence is the intelligent flow of awareness and insight that we experience once the mind and emotions are brought into balance and coherence through a self-initiated process. This form of intelligence is experienced as direct, intuitive knowing that manifests in thoughts and emotions that are beneficial for ourselves and others.

The HeartMath Solution provides a systematic way to consciously activate and develop this heart intelligence. With that solution, we can learn to expand our awareness and bring new coherence to our lives. In short, we can go beyond the brain.

## Early Exploration of the Heart

When I (Doc) founded the Institute of HeartMath in 1991, my colleagues and I embarked upon an in-depth study of the literature and research published on the heart. Having experienced significant improvements in our own lives through the practice of listening to and following our hearts, we turned our curiosity to the investigation of *how* and *why* that process works. We asked ourselves, "Does the heart operate simply under the direction of the brain, or does it possess an intelligence of sorts that has influence on our mind and emotions?" We wanted to understand how the physical heart communicates with the body and how it influences our whole system.

Although the words "heart" and "math" are rarely used together, I felt that this thought-provoking combination reflected the two most essential aspects of our work. The word "heart" has meaning to almost everyone, of course. When we think of "heart," we think of the physical heart as well as qualities such as wisdom, love, compassion, courage, and strength—the higher aspects of all human beings. The word "math" resonates with most people as well. In the context of

"HeartMath," it refers to the stepping stones of the system—the nuts-and-bolts approach to systematically unfolding "heart" qualities. It also refers to physiological and psychological equations for accessing and developing the incredible potential of the heart. The term "HeartMath" thus represents the importance of both fire and precision in our exploration of the heart.

For centuries, poets and philosophers have sensed that the heart is at the center of our lives. Saint-Exupéry, perhaps the most spontaneously boyish author of our time, wrote, "And now here is my secret, a very simple secret; it is only with the heart that one can see rightly; what is essential is invisible to the eye." [2]

The world's languages are filled with idioms about the heart. We use them to express our instinctive knowledge that the heart is the source of our higher qualities. When people are sincere, we often say that they're "speaking from the heart." When they throw themselves into an activity, we say that they're doing it "with all their heart." When people betray their own best interests, we comment that they're "thinking with their head, not their heart." And when they fall into despair, we worry that they've "become disheartened." Even our gestures indicate the importance we give to the heart: when people point to themselves, they generally point toward the heart.

In our explorations, we paid close attention to what had been written and said about the heart throughout history, wondering if there was more to this word "heart" than mere metaphor. If our culture were the only one to use the heart as a metaphor for high-quality feelings, we could consider it nothing more than a provincial turn of phrase, passed down through our ancestors. But over the centuries, the heart has been spoken of as a source of wisdom and feeling in almost all cultures. And many religions refer to the heart as the seat of the soul or the connecting place between spirit and humanness.

One of the observations that intrigued us most is that, throughout the ages, the heart has been referred to as a source not only of virtue but also of intelligence. The role of the heart as an intelligence within the human system is one of the most prevalent themes in ancient traditions and in inspirational writing. Blaise Pascal stated, "We know the truth not only by reason, but also by the heart." Lord Chesterfield wrote, "The heart has such an influence over the understanding that it is worth while to engage it in our interest." And Thomas Carlyle concluded, "It is the heart that always sees, before the head can see."

Many ancient cultures, including the Mesopotamians, the Egyptians, the Babylonians, and the Greeks, maintained that the primary organ capable of influencing and directing our emotions, our morality, and our decision-making ability was the heart; and they consequently attached enormous emotional and moral significance to its behavior.

Similar perspectives are found in the Hebrew and Christian bibles as well as in Chinese, Hindu, and Islamic traditions. The Old Testament saying in Proverbs 23:7, "For as a man thinketh in his heart, so is he," is further developed in the New Testament in Luke 5:22, "What reason ye in your hearts?"; these are but two examples. And in ancient Judaic tradition, the heart center, one of the *Sefirot* (energy centers) is known as *Tiffer et* (beauty, harmony, balance).

In the Kabbalah the heart is the Central Sphere, the only one of ten to touch all the others, and it's reputed to hold the key to the mysteries of radiant health, joy, and well-being. The aspect of balance and the attainment of bodily equilibrium is also attributed to the heart in Yogic traditions, which recognize the heart as the seat of individual consciousness, the center of life. In Yogic practice, the physical heart is considered both literally and figuratively the guide or internal "guru," and to this end, many Yogic practices cultivate an awareness of one's own heartbeat.

In traditional Chinese medicine, the heart is seen as the seat of connection between the mind and the body, forming a bridge between the two. It's said that the heart-blood houses the *shen*, which can be translated as both "mind" and "spirit." Thus the mind or spirit is housed in the heart, and the blood vessels are the communication channels that carry the heart's vital rhythmic messages throughout the body, keeping everything working in synchrony. It isn't surprising, then, that Chinese medicine holds that the state of each bodily organ as well as the body's integral functioning as a whole can be assessed via the pulse of the heart.

Whereas in the West, thought is seen as exclusively a function of the brain, the Chinese language itself represents a different perspective. The Chinese characters for "thinking," "thought," "intent," "listen," "virtue," and "love" all include the character for "heart." An ancient Chinese dictionary describes "silk threads" that connect the brain and heart. In the Japanese language there are two distinct words to describe the heart: *shinzu* denotes the physical organ, while *kokoro* refers to the "mind of the heart."[2a]

All these conceptions have a common view of the heart as harboring an "intelligence" that operates independent of the brain yet in communication with it. Are all of the cultures that share this view simply incorrect, perhaps not scientifically sophisticated enough to understand intelligence?

## A New Understanding of the Heart

Despite the colorful heart metaphors that enrich the many languages of the world, most of us have been taught that the heart is just a ten-ounce muscle that pumps blood and maintains circulation until we die. When something goes wrong, you hire a technician (called a doctor) to repair the organ. If worse comes to worst, you replace your pump with another one from someone who just died. This biological view sees the heart as a working part—one devoid of independent intelligence or emotion.

Looked at biologically, the heart's efficiency is amazing. The heart works without interruption for seventy to eighty years, without care or cleaning, without repair or replacement. Over a period of seventy years, it beats one hundred thousand times a day, approximately forty million times a year—nearly three billion pulsations all told. It pumps two gallons of blood per minute—well over one hundred gallons per hour—through a vascular system about sixty thousand miles in length (over two times the circumference of the earth). [3]

The heart starts beating in the unborn fetus before the brain has been formed. Scientists still don't know exactly what triggers the beating, but they use the word "autorhythmic" to indicate that the heartbeat is self-initiated from within the heart.

As the brain begins to develop, it grows from the bottom up. Starting from the most primitive part of the brain (the brainstem), the emotional centers (the amygdala and the hippocampus) begin to emerge. It is well known to brain researchers that the thinking brain then grows out of the emotional regions. That speaks volumes about the relationship of thought to feeling. In an unborn child there's an emotional brain long before there's a rational one, and a beating heart before either.

While the source of the heartbeat is within the heart itself, the timing of the beat is thought to be controlled by the brain through the autonomic nervous system. But surprisingly enough, the heart doesn't need a hardwired connection to the brain to keep beating. For example, when someone has a heart transplant, the nerves that run from the brain to the heart are severed, and surgeons don't yet know how to reconnect them. But that doesn't stop the heart from functioning. After surgeons have implanted a heart and restored its beat in a new person's chest, the heart keeps beating—though there's no longer any connection to the brain.

# The Brain in the Heart

In recent years, neuroscientists have made an exciting discovery. They've found that the heart has its own independent nervous system—a complex system referred to as "the brain in the heart." There are at least forty thousand neurons (nerve cells) in the heart—as many as are found in various subcortical centers in the brain. [4] The heart's intrinsic brain and nervous system relay information back to the brain in the cranium, creating a two-way communication system between heart and brain. The signals sent from the heart to the brain affect many areas and functions in the amygdala, the thalamus, and the cortex.

The amygdala is an almond-shaped structure deep inside the brain's emotional processing system. It specializes in strong emotional memories. The cortex is where learning and reasoning occur. It helps us solve problems and determine right from wrong. The amygdala, the thalamus, and the cortex work closely together. When new information comes in, the amygdala assesses it for emotional significance. It looks for associations, comparing what's familiar in emotional memory with this new information coming into the brain. Then it communicates with the cortex to determine what actions would be appropriate. [5]

The discovery that the heart has its own nervous system—a "brain" that affects the amygdala, the thalamus, and the cortex—helps to explain what physiologists John and Beatrice Lacey of the Fels Research Institute realized in the 1970s. At that time, it was known that the body's nervous system connected the heart with the brain, but scientists presumed that the brain made all the decisions. The Laceys' research showed that something else was happening.

The Laceys found that when the brain sent "orders" to the heart through the nervous system, the heart didn't automatically obey. Instead, the heart responded as if it had its own distinctive logic. Sometimes when the brain sent an arousal signal to the body in response to stimuli, the heartbeat sped up accordingly. But frequently it actually slowed down while the other organs responded with arousal. The selectivity of the heart's response indicated that it wasn't merely mechanically responding to a signal from the brain. Rather, the heart's response appeared to depend on the nature of the particular task at hand *and the type of mental processing it required*.

Even more intriguing, the Laceys found that the heart appeared to be sending messages back to the brain that the brain not only understood but obeyed. And it looked as though these messages from the heart could actually influence a person's behavior. [6]

The Laceys and others discovered that our heartbeats aren't just the mechanical throbs of a diligent pump, but an *intelligent language* that significantly influences how we perceive and react to the world. Subsequent researchers also discovered that the rhythmic beating patterns of the heart are transformed into neural impulses that directly affect the electrical activity of the higher brain centers—those involved in cognitive and emotional processing. [7–9]

In the 1970s, the Laceys' ideas were considered controversial. Yet even then, forward-looking thinkers glimpsed the depth and scope of these implications about the heart. In 1977, Dr. Francis Waldrop, then director of the National Institute of Mental Health, stated in a review article of the Laceys' work that "in the long run, their research may tell us much about what makes each of us a whole person and may suggest techniques that can restore a distressed person to health." [10]

One of our goals, as we pursued the HeartMath Solution, was to take the Laceys' work still further. They had established the heart's capacity to (in effect) "think for itself" under certain circumstances. We wanted to understand how the heart formulates its logic and influences behavior.

## What Is Intelligence?

For decades researchers have sought to understand the nature of intelligence. The first IQ tests were designed early in this century to measure intelligence as cognitive ability and intellect, and our school systems were geared up to help people develop both. Because it was found that IQ scores didn't increase much between kindergarten and adulthood, no matter how much education people received, many IQ experts argued that intelligence is inherited and can't be changed. They endorsed widely different estimates of the heritability of intelligence, ranging from 40 percent to 80 percent. [11]

Then in 1985 Howard Gardner published his research on "multiple intelligences" in his book *Frames of Mind*, which challenged our assumptions about intelligence. Gardner determined that intelligence is far more than mere intellect. He argued that the human system has many types of independent intelligences, including logical-mathematical, spatial, musical, bodily/kinesthetic, intrapersonal (dealing with self-knowledge), and interpersonal (dealing with knowledge of others). Gardner's research caused many people to reconsider the traditional view of intelligence as a one-dimensional construct and to think in new ways about the factors that determine personal, social, and professional success. [12] His discoveries stimulated educators to write new curricula to help children learn through their dominant intelligence. For example, children with high bodily/kinesthetic intelligence are taught math using physical games and movements to increase learning ability, comprehension, and retention.

Later in the 1980s John Mayer, a University of New Hampshire psychologist, and Peter Salovey of Yale co-formulated a new theory of "emotional intelligence" that shapes the quality of our intrapersonal and interpersonal relationships. Mayer and Salovey's definition of emotional intelligence includes five domains: knowing one's emotions; managing one's emotions; motivating oneself; recognizing emotions in others; and handling relationships. [13] Developing emotional intelligence involves the self-awareness of "becoming aware of both our mood and our thoughts about our mood." [11]

Reuven Bar-On, a clinical psychologist and lecturer in medicine at the Tel Aviv University Medical School, coined the term "emotional quotient" (or "EQ") in 1985. Bar-On devoted more than fifteen years of research to developing a formal psychological survey that aims to measure people's emotional intelligence. Based on his research and results, Bar-On summarized the qualities that contribute to emotional intelligence as follows:

> It is thought that the more emotionally intelligent individuals are those who are able to recognize and express their emotions, who possess positive self regard and are able to actualize their potential capacities and lead fairly happy lives; they are able to understand the way others feel and are capable of making and maintaining mutually satisfying and responsible interpersonal relationships without becoming dependent on others; they are generally optimistic, flexible, realistic and are fairly successful in solving problems and coping with stress without losing control. [14]

In 1996 Daniel Goleman wrote his groundbreaking book *Emotional Intelligence*. Goleman's exhaustive research confirmed that success in life is based more on our ability to manage our emotions than on our intellectual capabilities and that a lack of success is more often than not due to our mismanagement of emotions. His research helps explain why many individuals with a high IQ falter in life while others with only a modest IQ do exceptionally well. According to Goleman, the good news about emotional intelligence is that, unlike IQ, it can be developed and increased throughout life.

In his book, Goleman says that the ABCs of emotional intelligence include "self-awareness, seeing the links between thoughts, feelings and reactions; knowing if thoughts or feelings are ruling a decision; seeing the consequences of alternative choices; and applying these insights to choices."

This level of keen perception is a tall order for most people. In our fast-paced lives today, how do we stop to figure all these subtle factors out? How can we find emotional intelligence in the thick of an argument or an important business negotiation—a high-stakes situation in which we must make choices quickly? And how can we increase emotional intelligence in our society as a whole? "The question," Goleman says, "is how can we bring intelligence to our emotions—and civility to our streets and caring to our communal life?" [11]

## Cultivating Heart Intelligence

The answer lies in cultivating heart intelligence. It's our theory that heart intelligence actually transfers intelligence to the emotions and instills the power of emotional management. In other words, heart intelligence is really the source of emotional intelligence. From our research at the Institute of HeartMath, we've concluded that *intelligence* and *intuition* are heightened when we learn to listen more deeply to our own heart. It's through learning how to decipher the messages we receive from our heart that we gain the keen perception needed to effectively manage our emotions in the midst of life's situations and challenges. The more we learn to listen to and follow our heart intelligence, the more educated, balanced, and coherent our emotions become.

Without the guiding influence of the heart, we easily fall prey to reactive emotions such as insecurity, anger, fear, and blame, as well as other energy-draining reactions and behaviors. It's this lack of emotional management that brings incivility to our homes and streets and a lack of caring to our interactions with others—not to mention illness and accelerated aging.

Early in the Institute's research, we observed that when negative emotions threw the nervous system out of balance, they created heart rhythms that appeared jagged and disordered. [15] It was easy to see that a chronic state of nervous system and cardiovascular imbalance would put stress on the heart and other organs that could potentially lead to serious health problems.

Positive emotions, by contrast, were found to increase order and balance in the nervous system and produce smooth, harmonious heart rhythms. But these harmonious and coherent rhythms did more than reduce stress; they actually enhanced people's ability to clearly perceive the world around them. In order to be able to study these positive effects further, we taught our research subjects techniques that enabled them to generate a state of inner balance and harmony *at will* in the laboratory. [9, 16, 17] These techniques form the core of the HeartMath Solution.

The techniques that you'll learn in this book have been tested on hundreds of people from all walks of life. Once the heart rhythms of these research subjects came into balance and harmony, we found that they consistently reported increased mental clarity and intuition. When their heart rhythms shifted, they gained new control over their perceptions; and by gaining control over their perceptions, they were able to reduce stress and increase their effectiveness.

As they continued to practice these techniques in their daily lives, they reported increased creativity, enhanced communication with others, and a richer emotional experience of the textures of life. They also found that in this more balanced and coherent state, their perception of problems or difficult situations often widened enough that new perspectives and solutions emerged.

After Institute of HeartMath's scientists had begun to get consistent results in the lab, they extended their experiments to the workplace. The subjects of these new studies were asked to apply HeartMath Solution techniques during stressful situations at work. The results showed that these subjects were able to generate the same harmonious heart rhythms and shifts in nervous system balance in the workplace as other subjects had in the lab. [17]

The long-term results were even more encouraging. As the workplace participants practiced activating balanced heart rhythms consistently in their daily lives, they began to report benefits that went beyond our expectations. They reported a greater capacity to *sustain* a positive perspective, balance their emotions, and access an intuitive flow day to day, even in the midst of challenges.

Their ability to sustain these changes was important. It suggested that participants were actually able to *retrain their systems* to operate in a state of greater harmony—physically, mentally, and emotionally.

The tools of the HeartMath Solution had allowed these research subjects to experience positive emotions at will. Even beyond that, though, they had changed the tenor of participants' lives by enabling a consistent experience of positive emotions. Instead of constantly reacting to circumstances, these people were helped by heart intelligence to make coherent sense of their lives.

As science continues to discover how people can harness and direct the coherent power of the heart, it offers tremendous hope that society can shift from disorder and chaos to a new era of coherence and quality living for all.

# How Does Heart Intelligence Work?

Throughout this book we'll present research studies that help to explain how and why heart intelligence works. In the laboratory, Institute scientists have found that when subjects focus in the heart area and activate a core heart feeling such as love, appreciation, or care, this focus immediately shifts their heart rhythms. When the rhythms become more coherent, a cascade of neural and biochemical events begins that affects virtually every organ in the body.

Core heart feelings affect both branches of the autonomic nervous system. They *reduce* the activity of the sympathetic nervous system (that branch of the system that speeds heart rate, constricts blood vessels, and stimulates the release of stress hormones) and *increase* the activity of the parasympathetic nervous system (that branch of the system that slows heart rate and relaxes the body's inner systems), thereby increasing its effectiveness. In addition, the balance between these two branches of the nervous system is enhanced so that they work together with increased efficiency. This collaboration results in diminished friction and wear and tear on the nerves and internal organs.

Positive emotions such as happiness, appreciation, compassion, care, and love not only change patterns of activity in the nervous system; they also reduce the production of the stress hormone cortisol. Since the same precursor hormone is used in the manufacture of both cortisol and the anti-aging hormone DHEA, when cortisol is reduced DHEA production is increased. This powerful hormone is known to have protective and regenerative effects on many of the body's systems, and is believed to counter many of the effects of aging. [18]

Experiencing care and compassion has been shown to boost levels of IgA, an important secretory antibody that's the immune system's first line of defense. [19] Increased IgA levels make us more resistant to infection and disease. Numerous studies have revealed that feeling loved and cared for, along with caring for others around us, actually plays a greater role in increasing our health and longevity than physical factors such as age, blood pressure, cholesterol, or smoking. [20–24]

Since the act of evoking heart intelligence has been shown to facilitate brain function, adjust balance in the autonomic nervous system, lower blood pressure, increase stress-relieving hormones, and increase immune responses, it shouldn't surprise us that our bodies experience a sensation of well-being clear down to the cellular level—a sensation that we ourselves can induce. We feel better mentally and emotionally as a result of heart intelligence. And in the long run, that sensation translates into physical health. The best news of all is that these effects are attainable for each and every one of us.

We've been able to measure the impact of activating heart intelligence in employees of such large organizations as Motorola, Royal Dutch Shell, the IRS, the California Department of Justice, and the California Public Employees' Retirement System (CalPERS). After several weeks of learning how to access heart intelligence, these employees experienced a reduction in many common symptoms of stress—including rapid heart rate, sleeplessness, fatigue, tension, indigestion, and body aches. In one corporate study, blood pressure in hypertensive individuals was reduced to normal levels in just six months' time, without the aid of medication. [25]

Our case studies document clinical status improvements in people with various diseases and disorders, including arrhythmia, mitral valve prolapse, fatigue, autoimmune disorder, autonomic exhaustion, anxiety, depression, and post-traumatic stress disorder. [26, 27] In healthy individuals, significant positive shifts in hormonal balance have been measured in as little as one month. [18]

To achieve these results, we lead people through a process that teaches them how to gain access to the heart. In the training environment we customize that process, introducing the appropriate tools and techniques to fit specific needs. In this book we refer to a range of concepts, tools, and techniques used to activate heart intelligence as the HeartMath Solution. The following ten key tools and techniques govern the HeartMath Solution:

1. *Acknowledge your heart intelligence and its importance for making choices big and small.*

First, we need to gain a deeper understanding of the role the heart plays in health, perception, and overall well-being. Developing a new respect for the importance of the heart and grasping the significant influence it has over the rest of the body lays the foundation for understanding how and why the Heart-Math tools and techniques work.

The scientific evidence shared in these chapters also contributes to that foundation, showing how the heart communicates with the rest of the body and how information is exchanged between the heart and brain. As you come to understand the importance of this information exchange, you'll also realize why the core values and qualities long associated with the heart are important.

This first part of the learning process also involves discerning the difference between the head and the heart and observing how differently we perceive the world around us when we're in contact with heart intelligence. The head—that is, the brain or mind—operates in a linear, logical manner that serves us well in many situations but limits us in others. Sometimes we need more than analysis and logic to solve a problem or unravel a complex emotional issue. Heart intelligence provides an intuitive, direct knowingness that's an essential aspect of our overall intelligence. When heart intelligence is engaged, our awareness is expanded beyond linear, logical thinking. As a result, our perspective becomes more flexible, creative, and comprehensive.

For example, when two people in love are out walking in the park and get caught in a downpour, the rain is no big deal. It's just rain. They get wet, and they dry themselves off. The rain may even be fun. Because the lovers are connected in the heart, it's easy for them to accept this spontaneous event with a playful spirit.

But if the same couple is arguing, feeling frustrated, disconnected from the heart, their attitude when it starts raining is very different. Instead of being inconsequential, the rain, when seen from the head, is annoying, a further outlet for their frustration.

In this example there's a distinct difference in the couple's *perception* of the rain. Seen from the heart, the rain is a natural, spontaneous event. Seen from the head, it's a frustrating problem. When heart intelligence is engaged, we see stress-free solutions to problems.

Experiencing heart intelligence with continuity requires building a reliable partnership between the heart and the head—a partnership that starts when you learn how to distinguish between these two interactive but very different sources of intelligence and can tell when your thoughts and feelings are being directed by the heart and when they're not. Gaining a new respect for and trust in the heart leads to new possibilities and a sense of hope that we can break through and find solutions to our problems.

2. *Reduce stress.*

Biomedical research on internal coherence shows how detrimental stress is to humans. Internal coherence within an individual can be measured by monitoring the heart's rhythmic patterns. When a system is coherent, virtually no energy is wasted; power is maximized. Coherence is efficiency in action. Coherent people thrive mentally, emotionally, and physically. They have the power to adapt, to innovate. As a result, they experience little stress.

The net effects of increased internal coherence are significant: we spend less energy maintaining health, we waste less energy on inefficient thoughts and reactions, and we need not strain our body to keep focused and productive.

Stress is the enemy. It creates an incoherent internal state, pitting our biological systems against each other—which in turn affects how we think and feel. In the incoherence created by stress, our nervous system and heart rhythms become desynchronized and our hormonal balance is compromised. Consequently, incoherence diminishes our capacity to perform and to live a quality life, and it impacts our health negatively. Learning the value of coherence and the consequences of incoherence is crucial, because it provides sound reasoning for living a life directed by the heart.

3. *Learn and apply* FREEZE-FRAME.

FREEZE-FRAME is a simple, five-step technique that gives you access to core heart values and to the power of the heart to take you from incoherence to coherence. FREEZE-FRAME creates balance between the two branches of the autonomic nervous system, the sympathetic and the parasympathetic. The autonomic nervous system (ANS) interacts with our digestive, cardiovascular, immune, and hormonal systems. Negative mental and emotional responses such as anger and worry create disorder and imbalance in the ANS, while positive responses such as appreciation and compassion create increased order and balance. Increased order in turn results in more efficient brain function. By intentionally shifting into a more aware perceptual state through the FREEZE-FRAME technique, we modify input from the heart to the brain via the ANS.

FREEZE-FRAME is useful for making in-the-moment shifts in perception and attitude. When you need clarity to make decisions—big and small—or to reduce stress, use the FREEZE-FRAME technique.

Here's an example of how it works. Say you're at the office on a typically busy day. Everything is moving fast—but then things start to become confusing and chaotic. You feel so overloaded, so stressed out, that you don't know how to proceed. So you stop for sixty seconds and use FREEZE-FRAME to calm your mind, synchronize your nervous system, and increase your level of internal coherence. Then you see clearly your options for dealing with the situation. From the more balanced state of awareness that FREEZE-FRAME results in, you get a handle on how to do what needs to be done in less time with less stress. Simply said, FREEZE-FRAME helps to manage your thoughts and reactions and thereby reduces stress.

4. *Accumulate energy assets and decrease energy deficits.*

In this key step of the HeartMath Solution, you'll develop a new awareness of how effective you are at using your mental and emotional energy reserves. Our internal power—in other words, the amount of physical, mental, and emotional energy we have—is a determining factor in the quality of our lives. Internal power translates into vitality and resiliency.

Positive thoughts and feelings add energy to our system. An optimistic perspective, a feeling of appreciation, or a gesture of kindness, for example, are energy assets. Negative thoughts and feelings deplete our store of energy. Anger, jealousy, and judgmental thoughts, for example, are energy deficits.

By learning how to better observe our thoughts and feelings, our mental and emotional energy expenditures, we can identify where we're losing or gaining internal power. With this new awareness, we can begin to see where we need to make changes to increase that power. In Chapter 5 we'll introduce the concept of energy efficiency and give you a tool—the asset/deficit balance sheet—on which to record your mental and emotional energy expenditures.

5. *Activate core heart feelings.*

There are many core heart feelings, including love, compassion, nonjudgment, courage, patience, sincerity, forgiveness, appreciation, and care. All these feelings increase synchronization and coherence in the heart's rhythmic patterns. In the chapters to come, we'll focus on four key core heart feelings—appreciation, nonjudgment, forgiveness, and care (which are essential to the unfoldment of other core feelings).

Each core heart feeling has a powerful, beneficial effect on how you relate to life. Unfortunately, the experience of core heart feelings and attitudes is usually random rather than conscious. But you can cultivate core heart feelings, activating them on demand, to facilitate your personal growth and health.

6. *Manage your emotions.*

Emotions are complex and can be difficult to manage. It's essential that you do manage them, however, if you want to make your life rewarding and healthy. As you gain knowledge about your emotions—how they work, what effect they have, and how emotional integrity can be compromised—you'll learn how to better regulate them.

Emotions act as amplifiers of our thoughts, perceptions, and attitudes. We can have a great sound system with a state-of-the-art CD player and excellent speakers, but if the amplifier—the power source for our sound system—isn't working correctly, the sounds produced by the system are severely distorted. Likewise, when our emotions—the amplifiers of our perceptions—are out of balance, our view of life is distorted.

Positive emotional states are rewarding and regenerative to the heart, immune system, and hormonal system, while negative emotions drain these same systems. For most of us, every day is an emotional roller-coaster—sometimes we're up, sometimes we're down. Unless we consciously develop our ability to self-activate positive emotional states and arrest negative emotional states, we find it hard to stay balanced, healthy, and fulfilled. By learning about biomedical research on emotions, we can gain the ability to harness the power of emotion and use that power in ways that benefit rather than drain us.

7. *Care—but don't overcare.*

It's critical to learn the difference between care and overcare. Caring for yourself and others is an essential ingredient for a rewarding life. Unfortunately, caring can also be stressful. When our care goes too far, we experience what we call "overcare," a term that denotes a burdensome sense of responsibility accompanied by worry, anxiety, or insecurity. A host of problems result when we allow our care to become draining, including lowered immune response, imbalanced hormone levels, and poor decision-making. When we learn to distinguish between care and overcare, we're able to consciously choose the former and avoid the latter; we're empowered to stop taking our care—whether for people, things, or issues—to extremes. Once we recognize overcare and understand its ineffectiveness, we can begin to eliminate it from our thoughts and feelings. Understanding where and how you overcare will give you a new sense of freedom.

8. *Learn and apply* CUT-THRU.

The next major tool in the HeartMath Solution is CUT-THRU, a scientifically designed technique to help you manage your emotions and eliminate overcare.

Nonproductive thoughts are only as detrimental as the amount of emotion we add to them. For instance, we can have a sense of concern about an issue, but if we get really emotional about that issue, the concern can easily become anxiety or even panic. CUT-THRU will give you a reliable method to stop experiencing emotions that create incoherence and energy deficits.

By practicing the HeartMath Solution, you'll be able to clearly see when you're in stress. Then you can use FREEZE-FRAME to determine your best course of action. But even once you have intuitive clarity on what to do, you may still experience residues of uncomfortable or perplexing feelings. When those residues clog the system, you need to apply CUT-THRU, shifting your emotional state so that you're not only thinking better but also feeling better.

For many of us, long-standing emotional issues—feelings of betrayal, unworthiness, or fear, perhaps—color our lives in ways that block us from sustaining pleasurable emotional states. Applying the CUT-THRU technique to these emotional residues helps to dissolve and release them, even if they're deeply ingrained.

Institute of HeartMath research studies have demonstrated that CUT-THRU has a beneficial effect on hormonal balance, reduces unpleasant feeling states (such as anxiety, depression, guilt, and burnout), and increases positive feeling states (such as compassion, acceptance, and harmony).

This technique is a bit more complex than FREEZE-FRAME, but with practice it can be easily learned and applied in those areas of your life where more emotional management is needed.

9. *Do HEART LOCK-INS.*

The third major technique in the HeartMath Solution is the HEART LOCK-IN. Doing HEART LOCK-INS will amplify the power of your heart. Quieting the mind and sustaining a solid connection with the heart—*locking in* to its power—adds buoyancy and regenerative energy to your entire system. We'll share important research showing how the HEART LOCK-IN helps to sustain balance in your nervous system and improve immune system response.

HEART LOCK-INS, which take between five and fifteen minutes, strengthen the connection between heart and brain. Improving this connection makes it easier to stay in contact with your heart intelligence and its intuitive messages amidst your daily activities. Whereas FREEZE-FRAME is used to manage the mind and CUT-THRU to manage the emotions, HEART LOCK-IN is used to reinforce the practice of these other techniques and to activate a deeper connection with your core heart feelings and heart intelligence. Using the HEART LOCK-IN technique on a daily basis is beneficial for improving health, enhancing creativity, and experiencing more intuitive insight. You'll use HEART LOCK-IN as a tool to regenerate your system physically, mentally, and emotionally.

10. *Actualize what you know.*

The last step in the HeartMath Solution requires that you take all that you've learned from the first nine tools and techniques and apply that knowledge to different aspects of your life—personally, professionally, and socially. No matter what you're studying, application—*doing* what you know—is the most important part of the process. We'll share many examples of how others have used the HeartMath Solution to improve their personal lives, their health, and their families and organizations (including corporations, school systems, and government agencies). This information will give you insights into how the HeartMath Solution applies to your life and inspire you to practice the tools, techniques, and concepts you're learning.

To summarize, here's a psychological equation that clarifies the essence of the HeartMath Solution:

*Activating heart intelligence + managing the mind + managing the emotions = energy efficiency, increased coherence, enhanced awareness, and greater productivity*

With the right tools, living from the heart isn't as hard as it seems. After all, each of us has had experiences of the heart many times in our lives—and these experiences tend to be among our most enjoyable. However, they happen seemingly at random, and then they're gone. The HeartMath Solution will give you the ability to sustain a connection with your heart by teaching you to consciously listen to and follow your heart and to create heart-related experiences.

Melanie Trowbridge's story clearly illustrates the need for a systematic approach to living from the heart. Melanie was faced with a serious health challenge. After being diagnosed with ovarian cancer, Melanie went through six months of health problems including surgery, two bouts of pneumonia (with two long stays in the hospital), six two-day chemo treatments, and numerous days of nausea and weakness. It was a hard time, but everyone told her that she was handling the crisis extremely well—especially for someone who'd never been seriously ill before.

"I faced the crisis the only way I knew—by going to my heart for support as best I could. I felt better when I did that, but over time I either lost or began to ignore that connection to my heart. After the cancer went into remission and I started getting back into my 'normal' routine, I didn't listen as deeply to my heart as I had before. I began having extremely stressful fears that the cancer would return.

"When I attended a HeartMath seminar for professional reasons, I realized that during my health crisis I had followed my heart but hadn't known how to do it with consistency. I hadn't had a clue about what I was really doing! The HeartMath Solution tools and techniques gave me a way to stay connected with my heart intelligence, and the Institute of HeartMath's research clearly explained the importance of listening to it. I've felt more secure about the future of my health ever since."

Developing heart intelligence allows us to build a deep sense of inner security. People spend their lives looking for security outside themselves—in jobs, marriages, religions, and beliefs. Now there's a scientific approach to creating security within. As we develop a solid state of security in our hearts, we're able to do our jobs, enhance our marriages, and live our core values with more integrity.

## KEY POINTS TO REMEMBER

➤ Scientific evidence shows that the heart sends us emotional and intuitive signals to help govern our lives.

➤ Many ancient cultures maintained that the primary organ responsible for influencing and directing emotions, morality, and decision-making is the heart.

➤ The heart starts beating in an unborn fetus before the brain is formed. Scientists still don't know exactly what makes it start beating. The heartbeat is generated from within the heart itself and doesn't need a connection to the brain to keep beating.

➤ The heart has its own independent nervous system, referred to as "the brain in the heart." There are at least forty thousand neurons in the heart—as many as are found in various subcortical centers of the brain.

➤ Core heart feelings *reduce* the activity of the sympathetic nervous system (that branch of the system that speeds heart rate, constricts blood vessels, and stimulates the release of stress hormones in preparation for action) and *increase* the activity of the parasympathetic nervous system (that branch of the system that slows heart rate and relaxes the body's inner systems), thereby increasing its effectiveness.

➤ Positive emotions such as happiness, appreciation, compassion, care, and love improve hormonal balance and immune system response.

➤ From the research at the Institute of HeartMath, we've concluded that both intelligence and intuition are heightened when we learn to listen more deeply to our own hearts.

➤ There are ten key tools and techniques that make up the HeartMath Solution.

# CHAPTER 2

# The Ultimate Partnership

*proof that your heart and head can reach perfect harmony*

The intellect quickly reminds you what a great value the all-new Corolla is, giving you more car for less.

Ah, but the heart leaps to tell you that with Corolla's added power, safety features, and good looks, you'll be traveling like a dignitary.

Which goes to show you that even adversaries can come together for a common good.

(Toyota magazine ad, *Scientific American*, 1998)

At one of our seminars, a woman told us a classic story of head and heart. Years before, she'd entered into a business deal with her cousin, who'd always been successful. The deal looked like a sure thing, and she was excited about signing the papers as she drove to the bank.

But as she entered the bank, she began to have an uncomfortable feeling—a tightness in her chest and butterflies in her stomach. Something didn't feel right about signing this deal, but when she thought about it everything seemed in order, so she did it anyway.

Four years later she was still dealing with her financial losses and a host of legal problems resulting from that business decision. She told us that it was one of the worst decisions she'd ever made. "Why didn't I listen to my heart and check it out more before I signed?" she said with a sigh.

Nothing her mind was aware of as she contemplated the pending business deal gave her any reason for concern, but "in her heart" she sensed trouble. Like all of us, she'd grown up in a culture that places a high value on reason and tends to be skeptical of anything as "inconclusive" as intuition. On this occasion, though, reason simply wasn't enough. When she looked at the facts, her mind saw no reason to back away. Her heart, on the other hand, was picking up signals that her mind hadn't responded to. Had she taken both her heart and her head into consideration, she could have saved herself years of grief.

## Inner Teamwork

When we speak of the heart and head in these pages, we're using the terms as we might in casual conversation. In that context, we generally associate "head" with processes such as thought, imagery, memorization, planning, deduction, calculation, manipulation, and even occasionally self-punishment. We associate "heart" with what we might call "feeling qualities"—qualities such as care, love, wisdom, intuition, understanding, security, and appreciation. But keep in mind that we're talking not just about the physical head and heart but about the inner energies and attitudes *associated* with those areas of our bodies.

As scientists at the Institute of HeartMath (and others at the leading edge of neurocardiology research) continue to investigate the heart, we'll ultimately have a far greater understanding of the impact of the physical heart and brain on each other. Already the latest discoveries of these scientists have given us a radically new and different view of the role of the heart in the human system. But until more scientific research is in, we still must refer to the heart and head somewhat metaphorically when we describe their effects.

Both the heart and the head process information that governs our bodily functions, determines our attitudes and responses, and generally maintains our connection to the world around us. But their approach to that information and their interpretation of the facts is often quite different, one from the other.

The head—which, for our purposes, includes the brain and mind—operates in a linear, logical manner. Its primary functions are to analyze, memorize, compartmentalize, compare, and sort incoming messages from our senses and past experiences and transform that data into perceptions, thoughts, and emotions. The head also regulates many of our bodily functions.

The head decides what's good and what's bad, what's appropriate and what's inappropriate. It separates and divides, cataloging as it goes so that we can draw from past experiences to make sense of the present and ponder the future.

By accumulating and combining millions of partial truths and volumes of incomplete data, the head manages to put together somewhat cohesive patterns of reality. When we recognize patterns in our lives, we're able to make certain presumptions about the world that save us time and energy. Imagine what it would be like if when you went to work each day you had to relearn everything you needed to know to do your job. Clearly, life would be much more difficult and complex if we couldn't rely on patterns.

But that pattern-making ability, essential though it is, has drawbacks. The head can easily get locked into set patterns. Instead of seeing things from a fresh perspective, it can stubbornly presume that it "knows what it knows" about people, places, issues, and ourselves, blocking us from seeing and accepting new possibilities. When stubborn mind-sets rule, all new information we encounter must conform to the head's existing paradigm to be perceived as valid. At the survival level, maintaining a sense of order and stability is essential. But when we're trying to find new solutions to problems, or trying to develop new attitudes, behaviors, or perspectives, it can be a liability.

We're born with most of the neurons that we'll ever have in our brains, but the patterns in which these cells connect to one another develop and change throughout our lives. As we experience our environment and learn new skills, neurons connect in a web, or network, forming intricate ensembles—neural circuitry, as it were—that underlie our perceptions, memories, behaviors, and habits.

Remember what it was like the first time you tried to drive a car—especially if it was a stick shift? Yet for most of us it took only a little practice—maybe a week or two—before we could drive with one hand, change the radio station with the other, and talk to a friend all at the same time! We developed new circuits in the brain that enabled us to master the challenging task. And our circuitry is changing every day. The more we practice or repeat any action, the stronger the circuitry for that behavior becomes. As we reinforce the behavior, it eventually becomes automatic to us.

Just as physical skills such as driving, walking, or playing a sport become automatic through repetition, so do mental and emotional attitudes and behaviors. As we repeatedly engage in the same thoughts and feelings, the neural circuitry underlying these patterns is strengthened. In essence, our mental and emotional patterns become "hardwired"—locked—into our brain's circuitry.

This explains why our heads can be so stubborn at times and why strongly ingrained perceptions, emotions, and attitudes are so hard to change. [1]

The intelligence of the heart, on the other hand, processes information in a less linear, more intuitive and direct way. The heart isn't only *open* to new possibilities, it actively scans for them, ever seeking new, intuitive understanding. Ultimately, the head "knows" but the heart "understands." The heart operates in a more refined range of information-processing capability, and (as we'll demonstrate) it has a strong influence over how our brain functions.

The heart shows us the inherent core values in our lives and brings us closer to the sense of true security and belonging that we all crave. Heart intelligence is often accompanied by a solid, secure, and balanced feeling. Thus we can tell when we're in contact with the heart by how it feels. The intelligence of the heart acts as an impetus for what some scientists call *qualia* — our experience of the feelings and qualities of love, compassion, nonjudgment, tolerance, patience, and forgiveness. These qualities are often accompanied by a peaceful, clear state of awareness. When we're engaged with our hearts, the mind slows down and our thoughts become more rational and focused. The deductive process starts to coalesce into clarity and understanding. We feel more in control, and we perceive life from a more hopeful, optimistic perspective. As people practice the tools and techniques that harness heart intelligence, they begin to notice that they feel less caught up in their problems and in the hectic pace of daily activity. Their perspective encompasses a wider view.

We've seen many cases that illustrate the effectiveness of cultivating heart intelligence and emphasizing core values such as appreciation, care, sincerity, and authenticity in the workplace. In one such case, the Information Technology Services Division of a large state agency in California had initiated a host of changes to meet new challenges in the information services marketplace. The stress associated with these changes created an office environment of fragmentation, misperception, and miscommunication at many levels. Management took action and brought in a team of HeartMath consultants and trainers to deliver an Inner Quality Management training program to 117 employees. During this training initiative, the employees were educated in the important role that the heart plays, biologically and psychologically, in change management. They were given the HeartMath Solution tools and techniques to help them activate heart intelligence to bolster their sense of security and teamwork and to reduce their stress levels. Psychological tests were administered before and after the training program was completed to measure any changes in emotional stress and social attitudes. Physical symptoms of stress were also assessed.

By learning how to operate from their core heart feelings in the moment and in day-to-day interactions, participants enhanced their capacity to defuse personal and organizational stress. Results showed significant decreases in anger (20 percent), depression (26 percent), sadness (22 percent), and fatigue (24 percent)—and significant *increases* in peacefulness (23 percent) and vitality (10 percent)—after the HeartMath training. Stress symptoms were also significantly reduced, including anxiety (21 percent), sleeplessness (24 percent), and rapid heartbeats (19 percent). These individual improvements led to a more harmonious organizational change-implementation process. The key to achieving these results was getting the participants to learn to trust and utilize their heart intelligence by activating their core heart feelings to deal with challenging situations. [2] (See Figure 2.1.)

## Heart/Brain Communication

The love and care we feel in our hearts certainly transcends science, but we at the Institute of HeartMath have always felt that it's important to understand as much as possible about what takes place biologically when our hearts "come alive." If the heart is in fact intelligent, we want to know how it communicates its messages. Our search for answers to this question has led to exciting scientific discoveries, many of which will be presented in detail in the following pages.

In exploring the physiological mechanisms by which the heart communicates with the brain and body, Institute of HeartMath scientists asked questions such as these: Why do most people, regardless of race, culture, or nationality, experience the feeling or sensation of love and other emotions in the area of the heart? How do emotional states affect the heart, the autonomic nervous system, the brain, and the hormonal and immune systems? And how does the heart's information-processing system influence the body's other systems, including the brain?

What they found is that the heart communicates with the brain and the rest of the body in three ways for which there's solid scientific evidence: *neurologically* (through the transmission of nerve impulses), *biochemically* (through hormones and neurotransmitters), and *biophysically* (through pressure waves). In addition, growing scientific evidence suggests that the heart may communicate with the brain and body in a fourth way: *energetically* (through electromagnetic field inter-

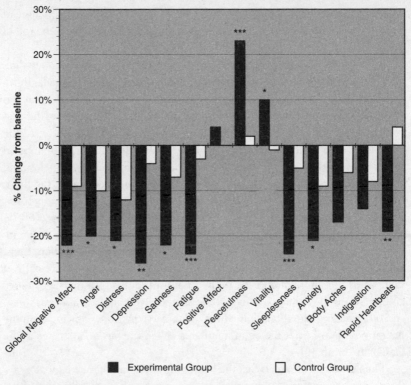

**Experimental Group** ☐ **Control Group**

***Emotional and Physical Health Improvements in Employees
Practicing the HeartMath Solution Tools and Techniques***

FIGURE 2.1. Only weeks after learning and practicing the tools and techniques of the Heart-Math Solution, the employees of a California state agency experienced significant reductions in stress, negative emotions, and fatigue; increases in peacefulness and vitality; and reductions in many common physical symptoms of stress (see black bars). A control group who didn't use the tools showed no significant changes (see white bars). *$p$ - .05, **$p$ - .01, ***$p$ - .001.

© copyright 1998 Institute of HeartMath Research Center

actions). Through these biological communication systems, the heart has a significant influence on the function of our brains and all our bodily systems. [3]

## Neurological Communication

In the last twenty years, a new discipline called *neurocardiology* has emerged. [4] It combines the study of the nervous system with the study of the heart.

Already this exciting new field is providing us with critical insights into some of the ways the brain and heart communicate with each other and with the rest of the body.

In 1991, after extensive research, one of the early pioneers in neurocardiology, Dr. J. Andrew Armour of Dalhousie University in Halifax, Canada, introduced evidence of a functional *heart brain*—the "brain in the heart" that was discussed briefly in Chapter 1. [5] From a neuroscience perspective, the nervous system within the heart is sufficiently sophisticated to qualify as a little brain in its own right. Dr. Armour's work has shown that this heart brain is an intricate network of several types of neurons, neurotransmitters, proteins, and support cells. Its elaborate circuitry allows it to act independent of the brain in the head. It can learn, remember, and even feel and sense. Through Dr. Armour's research, a very new picture of the heart has begun to emerge. [6]

With every beat of the heart, a burst of neural activity is relayed to the brain. The brain in the heart senses hormonal, rate, and pressure information, translates it into neurological impulses, and processes this information internally. It then sends the information back to the brain in the head via the vagus nerve and nerves in the spinal column. These same nerve pathways also carry pain and other feeling sensations to the brain. The nerve pathways flowing from the heart to the brain enter the brain in an area called the *medulla*, located at the base of the brain. [6]

The neurological signals that the heart sends the brain have a regulatory influence on many of the autonomic nervous system signals that flow out of the brain to the heart, to the blood vessels, and to other glands and organs. However, the signals that the heart sends the brain also cascade up into higher centers of the brain and influence the functioning of these centers. The work of the Laceys (discussed in Chapter 1), as well as that of other scientists after them, shows that neural messages from the heart affect the activity of the cortex—that part of the brain that governs our higher thought and reasoning capacities. [7–9]

The heart's input to the brain also influences neural activity in the amygdala (the important emotional center mentioned in Chapter 1). [10] Depending on the precise nature of the heart's input, it can at times inhibit, and at times facilitate, brain processes. [7–9, 11]

The heart also continuously influences our perceptions, emotions, and awareness. [3] The existence of communication pathways linking the heart with our higher brain centers helps explain how information from the heart can modify these mental and feeling states, as well as performance. Figure 2.2 provides a

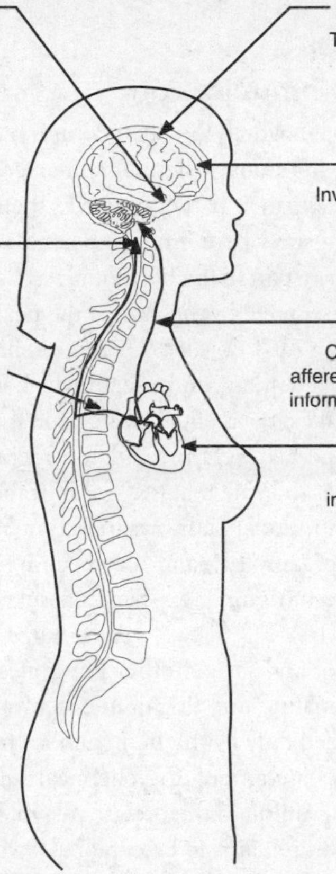

**Amygdala**

Storehouse of emotional memory – compares what's emotionally familiar with new incoming information

**Cerebral Cortex**

Thinks, strategizes, plans, reflects, inspires, and imagines

**Frontal Lobes**

Involved in decision-making – determine appropriate emotional responses

**Medulla**

Contains nerve centers that regulate breathing, heart rate, and other bodily functions

**Vagus Nerve**

Contains parasympathetic afferent nerve fibers that carry information from heart to brain

**Sympathetic Afferent Nerves**

Carry information from heart to brain through spinal cord

**Heart Brain**

Integrates and processes information from the heart, brain, and body

*Neurological Communication from the Heart to the Brain*

FIGURE 2.2. This diagram illustrates the neurological pathways through which the heart communicates with the brain. The heart's intrinsic nervous system (the *heart brain*) contains *sensory neurites* as well as *local circuit neurons* of several types. The sensory neurites, which are distributed throughout the heart, sense and respond to many types of biological information, including heart rate, pressure, hormones, and neurotransmitters. The local circuit neurons are arranged in processing stations that integrate inflowing neurological information from the brain and bodily organs with input from the heart's sensory neurites. Once the heart brain has processed this information, it sends messages to the brain via "afferent" neural pathways—that is, pathways that flow toward the brain. The *sympathetic afferent nerves* travel to the brain through the spinal cord. The *vagus nerve* contains thousands of nerve fibers, many of which also carry information from the heart to the brain. These neural pathways enter the brain in the *medulla,* a brain center that regulates many vital bodily functions. From there, the neurological information from the heart travels to higher brain centers involved in emotional processing, decision-making, and reasoning.

simplified illustration of the neurological communication pathways from the heart to the brain.

## Biochemical Communication

Another avenue through which the heart communicates with the brain and the rest of the body is the hormonal system. A *hormone* is defined as a chemical substance formed in one organ or part of the body, then carried in the bloodstream to another organ or tissue where it has a specific effect. In 1983 the heart was formally reclassified as a part of the hormonal system when a powerful new hormone produced and secreted by the atria of the heart was discovered. It's called *atrial natriuretic factor* (ANF) or *atrial peptide*. This hormone regulates blood pressure, body-fluid retention, and electrolyte homeostasis. Nicknamed the "balance hormone," it exerts its effects widely: on the blood vessels, the kidneys, the adrenal glands, and many of the regulatory regions of the brain. [12]

In addition, studies indicate that ANF inhibits the release of stress hormones [13], plays a part in hormonal pathways that stimulate the function and growth of our reproductive organs [14], and may even interact with the immune system. [15] Even more intriguing, experiments suggest that ANF can influence motivated behavior. [16]

In addition to ANF and several other hormones, the heart also synthesizes and releases noradrenaline and dopamine, neurotransmitters that were once thought to be produced only by the brain and in the ganglia outside the heart. [17] These molecules are among the chemical substances known to mediate emotion in the brain. Although the precise role of these neurotransmitters produced by the heart still remains to be explored, some scientists see their origin in the heart as another building block supporting the newly emerging view that the human "emotional system" isn't confined to the brain but is instead distributed in a network that extends throughout the entire body. [18] The heart is a central player in this network.

## Biophysical Communication

With every beat, the heart generates a powerful blood pressure wave that travels rapidly throughout the arteries, much faster than the actual flow of blood. It's these waves of pressure that create what we feel as our pulse.

Important rhythms exist in the oscillations of blood pressure waves. In healthy individuals a complex resonance occurs between blood pressure waves, respiration, and rhythms in the autonomic nervous system. [19] Because pressure-wave patterns vary with the rhythmic activity of the heart, they represent yet another language through which the heart communicates with the rest of the body. At the receiving end of the arteries are all the body's glands and organs. In essence, all of our cells "feel" the waves of pressure generated by the heart and are dependent on them in more than one way. At the most basic level, pressure waves force the blood cells through the capillaries and provide oxygen and nutrients to all our cells. In addition, these waves expand the arteries, causing them to generate a relatively large electrical voltage. The waves also apply pressure to the cells in a rhythmic fashion, causing some of the proteins contained therein to generate an electrical current in response to the "squeeze."

Experiments conducted at the Institute of HeartMath have shown that pressure waves are a biophysical means by which the heart communicates with the brain and influences its activity. In these investigations, researchers measured the timing of the arrival of the blood pressure wave at the brain while simultaneously measuring brain-wave activity. A change in the brain's electrical activity could be clearly seen when the blood pressure wave reached the brain cells. [3]

## Energetic Communication

As many doctors know, the pattern and quality of the energy emitted by the heart is transmitted throughout the body via the heart's electromagnetic field. Just as cell phones and radio stations transmit information via an electromagnetic field, recent research has led some scientists to propose that a similar information transfer process occurs via the electromagnetic field produced by the heart. [3, 20] The heart's electromagnetic field is by far the most powerful produced by the body; it's approximately five thousand times greater in strength than the field produced by the brain, for example. [20] The heart's field not only permeates every cell in the body but also radiates outside of us; it can be measured up to eight to ten feet away with sensitive detectors called *magnetometers*. (See Figure 2.3.)

Scientists at the Institute's laboratory and elsewhere have found that the electrical information patterns generated by the heart are detectable in our brain waves via a test known as an *electroencephalogram* (EEG). [20, 21] A series of experiments by Gary Schwartz and his colleagues at the University of Arizona found that the complex patterns of cardiac activity in our brain waves could not be fully explained by neurological or other established communication pathways. Their data provides evidence that there's a direct energetic interaction between the electromagnetic field produced by the heart and that produced by the brain. [20] Both Schwartz's research and that of the Institute of

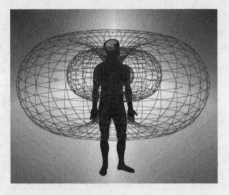

### The Heart's Electromagnetic Field

FIGURE 2.3. The electromagnetic field generated by the heart envelops the entire body and extends out in all directions into the space around us. The heart's electromagnetic field—by far the most powerful field produced by the body—can be measured many feet away from us by sensitive devices.

© copyright 1997 Institute of HeartMath Research Center

HeartMath demonstrate that when we focus attention on our hearts, the synchronization between our hearts and brains increases. Experiments suggest that the energetic interaction between the heart and brain plays a part in this process. [3, 20, 21]

Furthermore, research evidence indicates that energetic information contained in the heart's field isn't detected only by our own brains and bodies but can also be registered by the people around us. [3, 22] (You'll learn more about how this occurs in Chapter 8.)

## The Rhythm Master

The scientific research we've just reviewed clearly paints a picture of the heart as an intelligent system that processes many types of biological information independent of the brain. The neural, biochemical, biophysical, and electromagnetic messages that the heart generates and transmits to the brain and body have a profound influence on our physiological, mental, and emotional processes. But how do we decode these messages? Is there a scientific way to detect or measure what the heart is "saying" and to determine how this information affects our awareness at any given moment?

Over the years we've experimented with many different types of psychological and physiological measures. Heart rate variability (HRV) patterns, or heart rhythms, have consistently emerged as the most dynamic and reflective of our inner emotional states. *Heart rate variability* is defined as a measurement of beat-to-beat changes in the heart rate.

If you go to a doctor's office for a physical exam, she may tell you that your heart is beating at seventy beats per minute (bpm). This is only an average figure, of course, because the time interval between heartbeats is always changing. If the doctor takes your pulse with her fingertips—the usual method—she counts the total number of pulses within a certain period of time and you're unaware of any rate variation. If, on the other hand, you're attached to a heart rhythm monitor, you can actually observe the dramatic variation in heart rate that occurs even during inactivity.

Not more than thirty-five years ago, doctors thought that a steady heart rate was a sign of good health. But now, through HRV analysis, we know that it's normal for the heart rate to vary. In fact, the heart rate changes with every heartbeat even when we're asleep. Contrary to the earlier belief that a steady heart rate was an indicator of health, we now know that a loss of the naturally occurring variability in heart rate is actually a sign of disease and a strong predictor of future health problems.[23] Because heart rate variability declines as we get older, it's one way to measure our physiological aging.[24] In essence, HRV is a measure of the flexibility of our heart and nervous system, and as such reflects our health and fitness.

The Institute's research team was intrigued by HRV because changes in the rhythmic beating patterns of the heart hinted at a window into the inner workings of the communication pathways between the heart, brain, and body. It seemed possible that distinct patterns of neurological, biochemical, biophysical, and electromagnetic activity generated by precise variations in the timing between heartbeats could function as an intelligent language by which the heart conveyed meaningful information to the rest of the body. By measuring and analyzing HRV, the Institute's researchers began to see how the heart encodes its messages. Even more enticing was the discovery that these changing heart rhythms proved to be remarkably responsive to our thoughts and feelings. By measuring people's HRV, the research team was able to see how the heart and nervous system respond to stress and different emotions as we experience them. [25]

When we hook people up to a heart rhythm monitor during our seminars, people are amazed to see that the slightest emotional change shows up immediately in both a change in heart rate and a change in the HRV pattern. When a fairly calm business manager at one of our seminars was hooked up to the monitor, he started off with a low heart rate of 65 bpm and a relatively smooth HRV pattern. But as soon as someone in the class made a joke and he laughed, his heart rate bounced up to 94 bpm for several moments before settling back to its usual rate.

As he began to do the stressful exercise of counting backwards from two hundred by seventeens, his HRV pattern revealed that his heart was changing tempo erratically. (This same erratic pattern occurs when we feel stress from any frustration or anxiety.) But when he focused on his heart by appreciating someone he loved, his HRV quickly shifted to a smoothly ordered, coherent pattern. We could see that his heart was now speeding up and slowing down in a harmonious flow.

The analysis of HRV enables us to listen in on and interpret ongoing, two-way conversations between heart and brain. As we perceive and react to the world, messages sent by the brain through the autonomic nervous system affect the heart's beating patterns. At the same time, the heart's rhythmic activity generates neural signals that travel back to the brain, influencing our perceptions, mental processes, and feeling states.

As mentioned in Chapter 1, it became clear to us early on in our research that the experience of negative emotions—anger and frustration, for example—creates increased disorder and incoherence in the heart's rhythms and in the autonomic nervous system, thereby affecting the rest of the body. In contrast, positive emotions such as love, care, and appreciation create increased harmony, order, and coherence in the heart's rhythms and improved balance in the nervous system. Heart rate variability can be looked at as an important measurement of how well we're balancing our lives mentally and emotionally. [26]

The health implications are easy to understand: disharmony in our heart rhythms leads to inefficiency and increased stress on the heart and other organs, while harmonious rhythms are more efficient and less stressful to the body's systems.

The typical HRV pattern of someone feeling angry or frustrated looks irregular and disordered (Figure 2.4). The sympathetic and parasympathetic branches of the autonomic nervous system are out of sync with each other, battling for control over the heart rate—the sympathetic trying to speed it up and the parasympathetic trying to slow it down. It's as if you were trying to drive your car with one foot on the accelerator and the other simultaneously on the brake. Most of us value our cars too highly to treat them in this way—yet, without realizing it, we treat ourselves in this way more than we know.

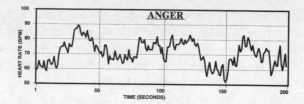

## Negative Emotions and Heart Rate Variability

FIGURE 2.4. In negative emotional states such as anger (pictured here) and frustration, the HRV pattern is incoherent, random, jerky. This indicates disharmony in the autonomic nervous system, which carries information from the brain to the heart and throughout the body.

© copyright 1998 Institute of HeartMath Research Center

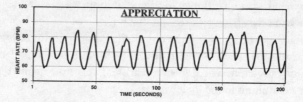

## Positive Emotions and Heart Rate Variability

FIGURE 2.5. In positive emotional states such as appreciation (pictured here), love, and care, the HRV pattern is coherent and ordered. Such a pattern is generally associated with autonomic nervous system balance and cardiovascular efficiency.

© copyright 1998 Institute of HeartMath Research Center

When we feel edgy or stressful, we create a disordered heart rhythm. This creates a chain reaction in our bodies: our blood vessels constrict, our blood pressure rises, and a lot of energy is wasted. If this happens consistently, the result is hypertension (high blood pressure), which greatly increases the risk of heart disease and stroke. It's now estimated that one in four Americans—approximately fifty million people—are hypertensive, and cardiovascular disease now claims more lives each year in the United States than the next seven leading causes of death combined. [27]

The good news is that feelings of appreciation, love, compassion, and care create the opposite effect. These positive heart-based feelings generate the smooth and harmonious HRV rhythms that are considered to be indicators of cardiovascular efficiency and nervous system balance (Figure 2.5).

When we're generating positive feelings, the two branches of the nervous system are in sync, working in harmony. And that's good news for our health. As we'll see in later chapters, creating increased order in the autonomic nervous system produces beneficial effects throughout the body—including enhanced immunity [28, 29] and improved hormonal balance. [30]

## Entrainment

In the seventeenth century, a European inventor by the name of Christiaan Huygens took great pride in his invention of the pendulum clock. He maintained a fine collection of such clocks in his studio. One day, when he was in bed, he noticed a peculiar thing: all the pendulums were swinging in unison, though he knew they hadn't started out that way.

Christiaan got out of bed and started all the pendulums swinging differently, breaking the synchronized rhythm. To his amazement, all the pendulums soon fell back into synchronization again. Every time he misaligned their swing, the pendulums found their way back into sync.

Although Christiaan couldn't completely solve the mystery, later scientists did: the largest pendulum—the one with the strongest rhythm—was pulling the other pendulums into sync with it. This phenomenon, termed *entrainment*, has been found to be prevalent throughout nature (Figure 2.6). [31]

When your body is in entrainment, its major systems work in harmony. Your biological systems operate at higher efficiency because of that harmony, and as a result you think and feel better. Because the heart is the strongest biological oscillator in the human system—the equivalent of the strongest pendulum in a collection of clocks—the rest of the body's systems can be pulled into entrainment with the heart's rhythms. As an example, when we're in a state of deep love or appreciation, the brain synchronizes—comes into harmony—with the heart's harmonious rhythms, as shown in Figure 2.7. [3, 21] This state of head/heart entrainment occurs precisely when the heart rhythms complete one cycle every ten seconds (0.1 Hz).

When brain waves entrain with heart rhythms at 0.1 Hz, subjects in our studies report heightened intuitive clarity and a greater sense of well-being. HeartMath's FREEZE-FRAME, CUT-THRU, and HEART LOCK-IN techniques (which we'll address in Chapters 4, 9, and 10) are designed to help people get their heads and hearts in sync. These techniques work precisely because they encourage a coherent state of entrainment.

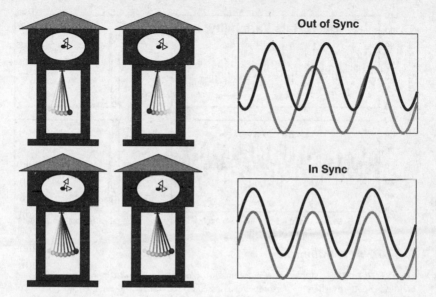

*Entrainment*

FIGURE 2.6. When two pendulum clocks are mounted side by side on the same wall, they gradually come to swing in synchrony. In this state, the clocks generate the wave pattern shown in the bottom right-hand panel. This is a classic example of the phenomenon of *entrainment*, which occurs throughout nature (both in nonliving systems and in living organisms). In general, when systems entrain, they operate with increased efficiency. In the human body, the heart—as the body's most powerful rhythmic oscillator—is the central "pendulum" that sets the stage for entrainment of other physiological systems.

According to our studies, at those elusive moments when we transcend our ordinary performance and feel in harmony with *something else*—whether it's a glorious sunset, inspiring music, or another human being—what we're really coming into sync with is *ourselves*. Not only do we feel more relaxed and at peace at such moments, but the entrained state increases our ability to perform well and offers numerous health benefits. In entrainment, we're at our optimal functioning capacity.

Our research shows that people can develop their ability to maintain entrainment by sustaining sincere, heart-focused states such as appreciation and love. The results of studies on head/heart entrainment suggest that by intentionally altering our emotional state through specific techniques, we modify the

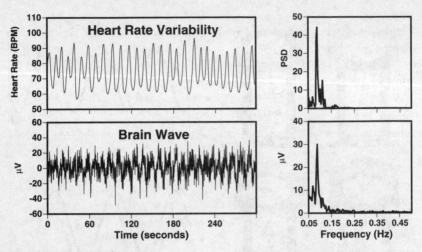

*Head/Heart Entrainment*

FIGURE 2.7. These graphs show entrainment occurring between heart rate variability and brain-wave patterns when the person being assessed FREEZE-FRAMED and experienced a feeling of sincere appreciation. The left-hand graphs show the real-time recordings of the person's heart rhythms and brain waves. The right-hand graphs show the frequency spectra of the same data. Notice how the heart rhythms and brain waves have synchronized at a frequency of approximately 0.1 Hz (large spike in right-hand graphs) during FREEZE-FRAME.

© copyright 1998 Institute of HeartMath Research Center

input from the heart to the brain. Our bodies were designed to function at optimum capacity when the heart and head are highly attuned to one another and working together.

## Let's Make a Deal

The preceding scientific information provides solid evidence that in fact the heart does communicate many messages to the brain. But what do we experience when we learn to refine and heighten that communication from heart to head?

The challenge in maximizing the heart's influence on the brain lies in getting the head to surrender to the heart long enough to connect with heart intelligence—and it often puts up a real fight! No matter how valuable the heart's input may be, it often disrupts the brain's familiar mode of operation. When old neurological patterns ingrained through years of habit are challenged, they sometimes hold on for dear life.

If the heart sends a clear intuitive signal with a feeling that says, "Don't do this!" the head may vigorously resist, demanding to know "Why?" "How?" and "When?" so persistently that the heart's signal is cut off. You might have a major insight about behavior you need to change, for example, but before you have a chance to transform that insight into action, you begin to think of justifications and rationalizations that persuade you not to change.

Sally got upset every time she heard her sister, Linda, and Linda's husband get into an argument. Before she knew it, Sally would join the fray, mediating and offering advice, and then all three of them would end up arguing.

Feeling misunderstood and hurt, Sally would leave their house vowing never to get involved again. Each time it happened, she stayed upset for days, analyzing and dwelling on what she should have said differently.

Many times, as an argument was starting, the intuition from her heart would tell Sally to stay out of it. But her head would immediately counter with reasons for involvement: "Linda is my sister. I love her and can't stand to see her hurt like this. She needs my help." This process went on for years—the head winning out each time—making Sally miserable.

If Sally had had the HeartMath Solution tools and techniques at her disposal, she would have been able to make a solid connection between her heart and her head; and with that connection she would have understood more clearly the wisdom of her heart. From that more integrated perspective, she would have been able to express her love for her sister and brother-in-law without getting emotionally involved in their problems.

Most of us can think of times when we've had a clear intuition from the heart about what to do (or not do) but have overanalyzed the situation, going around and around in an attempt to figure things out. In Sally's case, circumstances played on her emotions—the love she felt for her sister and her own anxiety over the pain they seemed to be causing one another. But instead of letting her heart increase her awareness, Sally's head engaged in an "intelligence reduction process," keeping her from seeing other options.

The head often leads us into rationalizing and conceptualizing an issue instead of actualizing what the heart already knows and has communicated. When we react to life from the head without joining forces with the heart, our single-mindedness often leads us into childish, inelegant behavior that we're ashamed of. If, on the other hand, we get the head in sync with the heart, we have the power of their teamwork on our side and can make the changes we know we ought to make.

## Higher Heart, Lower Heart

W ait a minute," you might say. "I've followed my heart before and gotten hurt, stepped on, and screwed." That's certainly a common experience. You trust someone, believing that he cares for you as you care for him, only to discover that he's out for himself—at your expense. This type of realization is so common, in fact, that learning to handle the shock of it with grace is one of the rites of passage to adulthood.

With experience, we begin to anticipate betrayal sooner and soften its blow. But inside, many people look back on early painful events with a bitterness that's toxic and self-destructive. Believing that their vulnerability and care got them hurt, they cut themselves off from spontaneous expression of the heart. They become guarded and slow to love again. "My heart got me into this," they think.

The ability to protect ourselves from pain is an important survival mechanism. But cutting off the heart is a misguided defensiveness grounded in the belief that following the heart means following our emotions—a belief that's just not true. The fact that we feel something strongly—anger or fear or desire— doesn't mean that the emotion is driven by the heart. In fact, the head often uses emotional backup to get its own way, hijacking our emotions to defend its fears, projections, and desires whether they're aligned with heart intelligence or not.

When we're first learning to make the distinction between the head and the heart, it's easy to be fooled. But there's a big difference between emotions driven by the head and emotions of the true heart. To avoid confusion, we like to speak of emotions in terms of the "higher" and "lower" heart.

The lower heart refers to those feelings that are colored by the attachments and conditions placed on them by the mind. Conditional love is a good example: "I'll love you as long as you do things I like." The heart wants to give, but the mind wants to renege, to hedge its bets and get what it wants.

The higher heart is more allowing. It doesn't hedge or barter. Instead of saying, "I'll do this *if* you do that," it expresses itself authentically without expectation. Authenticity is its own reward for the higher heart. But it takes emotional maturity to manifest the heart's qualities with consistency.

Take the feeling of sympathy, for example. It certainly seems admirable at first glance. When a friend says her life has gone to hell and gives supporting evidence, quite naturally you feel sympathetic. Then you start agonizing on her behalf. What could be wrong with that? But think about it. How do you feel after spending time with her? Exhausted? Depleted? In need of a break? The sympathetic "bleeding heart" is lower heart. Feeling what another feels is admirable, but we need to exercise caution in expressing our empathetic feelings and caring intentions.

We've noticed in our own lives that too much sympathy isn't helpful. It's draining—and to no useful end. Sympathy kicks in when our heads overidentify with someone in need and we start projecting our own concerns. Our heads persuade us that in order to be a good friend, we have to "get into" that person's pain, identify with it and make it our own. But that means engulfing ourselves in the same draining emotions our friend is suffering from. By the time we project our own concerns about the problem on top of our friend's concerns, we're sinking into an emotional bog that's not helpful to anyone. That's why an offer of sympathy so often leads to two people crying in their beers instead of one—with no solution in sight.

Compassion, on the other hand, is regenerative, and it offers intuitive understanding and potential solutions. It lets us feel what another is feeling while holding on to our own authenticity. We can embrace our suffering friend without falling into over-responsibility and despair. Caring about the problems and concerns of those we love is a natural part of friendship. We just need to make sure that our feelings of care lead to higher-heart compassion rather than lower-heart sympathy.

Because we don't usually make a distinction between higher and lower heart, we tend not to notice the difference, lumping both sorts of emotions together in the "heart" category. Think back on the last time you gave your heart to someone and got hurt. Can you tell, with the wisdom of hindsight, which kind of heart you were feeling? Were you following your true heart, or were you responding to an amalgam of head expectations, lower-heart emotions, and heart feelings? Was the pain caused by the love you felt or by unmet hopes and conditions?

When we learn to manage our emotions long enough to stop and shift our attention to the quieter message of the heart, we can gain a wider perspective on any situation, often saving ourselves from hurt, frustration, and pain.

When I (Howard) was twenty-one, I discovered firsthand just how hard finding the true heart can be. Out of the blue, my girlfriend left me for a more mature (and much richer) man. I was totally blindsided by her defection. We'd been together for four years when she sent me her "Dear Howard" letter. My heart was broken. I went into shock, distraught with hurt, remorse, embarrassment, and despair. When I found out that two of my friends had been encouraging the new relationship behind my back, I added anger and revenge to my growing list of brokenhearted emotions.

In this emotionally distorted state, I decided that because I really loved her I should try to win her back. After all, she was *my girl*; I wasn't going to let some hotshot walk away with her without putting up a fight. I arranged to see her and we had "the talk," both of us feeling the pull of our emotional history. In a moment of intense emotional connection, I asked her to marry me. She was touched deeply by my expression of commitment and went away to think about the proposal. I had really followed my heart this time—or so I thought.

The next day when Doc showed up, I proudly told him what I'd done. To my surprise, Doc's take on the situation was a little different from mine—to say the least. He said that the part of me that was feeling broken wasn't my heart, wasn't the real essence of love I felt for her. It was my attachments and expectations that were broken, and this damage was fueling my insecurities. He went on to suggest that the real act of love I should show her was to contact her again and release her from the marriage proposal.

"If she comes back on her own," he said, "you've got something solid and clean to build on. If she doesn't, you've still done the most loving thing you could do in this situation, and somewhere along the way that will pay off. You'll just have to pick up the pieces and move on, but it can only be through letting her have the freedom she needs to make her decision that you'd really be loving her."

That was about the last thing I wanted to hear, but hear it I did. I'd read about the concept of unconditional love, but this was real, not conceptual. It was hard to do because of the love I felt for her—but at the same time it made sense to strive for a higher form of love rather than one based on my own insecurity and hurt feelings. For several hours after Doc left, my head and my heart engaged in battle. Eventually, though, the heart won out. I made the call and gave her an unconditional release. She didn't come back to me; she married the other man and to my knowledge is still happily married to him.

Although I didn't feel a sense of resolution, peace, or release immediately, I did experience a feeling of empowerment that gave me a sense of security and self-confidence. Over time that gift grew in value and enabled me to love in a whole new way. I went on with my life, easily found new and rewarding relationships, and today I'm more than happily married myself.

What looks like heart often isn't the real McCoy. And what the real heart tells us often isn't what the head wants to hear. The head is motivated by quick results, so it gets discouraged if the heart's rewards are slow to show up. Despite these challenges, however, listening to your heart—with its deeper insight and intuitive understanding—is always the wisest course of action.

The Institute's research, as well as the research of others, has revealed that knowing how things work can deeply enhance our appreciation of them. As Dr. Mark George, lead psychiatrist at the Medical University of South Carolina, points out, "If I understand . . . all there is to know about the sound coming from a violin, striking my ear and then going into my brain, this does not detract from the joy of a well-played symphony. Knowing mechanisms does not take away from the joy of experience and often adds yet another dimension." [32]

It's the same with the science of the heart. When it comes to the bottom line—how we live and experience our lives—the most important aspect of heart intelligence is that it *works*, that when you put it into practice, you maximize your own potential for health and well-being. We don't need science in order to listen to our hearts. People have been doing it for ages. But in an effort to enhance our experience and appreciation of heart intelligence, we can look to science to help us understand how it works.

It's easier than you might think to listen to the signals and messages of the heart. We're naturally wired for this communication. Right down to the biological level, the components for the ultimate partnership already exist.

We've all heard the voice of our heart before, whether we followed it or not. As we learn more about the heart and find that we can trust its contributions to our awareness, a new and more rewarding life experience will emerge for us, both as individuals and as a society. Given that potential payoff, following the heart is certainly worth considering. After all, a life without heart just isn't much fun.

## KEY POINTS TO REMEMBER

> New scientific discoveries are giving us a radically new and different view of the role of the heart in the human system.

➢ Information sent from the heart to the brain can have profound effects on our higher brain centers.

➢ Our emotional states are reflected in our heart rhythms, as seen in heart rate variability measurements. Our heart rhythms affect the brain's ability to process information, make decisions, solve problems, and experience and express creativity.

➢ Because the heart is the strongest biological oscillator in the human system, the rest of the body's systems are pulled into entrainment with the heart's rhythms.

➢ When subjects in research studies achieve entrainment of the brain with the heart, they report heightened intuitive clarity and a greater sense of well-being.

➢ Positive feelings such as appreciation create increased order and balance in the autonomic nervous system, resulting in enhanced immunity, improved hormonal balance, and more efficient brain function.

➢ By intentionally altering our emotional state through heart-focused techniques such as FREEZE-FRAME, we modify input from the heart to the brain. The changed information flow from the heart to the brain can facilitate higher brain function.

➢ When we get the head in sync with the heart, the power of both works for us and we can make changes that we know we ought to make.

➢ The so-called lower heart governs feelings that are colored by attachments and conditions placed on them by the mind.

PART 2

# Accessing Heart Intelligence

Now that we appreciate the importance of heart intelligence and understand how it works biologically, it's time to learn how to systematically access it.

In Part II we'll first discuss what blocks us from heart intelligence and then look at what we can do to eliminate these obstacles to create a reliable partnership between head and heart.

A primary goal of the HeartMath Solution is to increase coherence, bringing us to a state of optimal efficiency. Stress creates incoherence in our system, so *increasing* coherence necessitates *reducing* stress. In the chapter that follows, we'll spell out the perils of stress.

Then, once we've emphasized how draining stress is—and how crucial it is to eliminate it—we'll introduce the FREEZE-FRAME technique in Chapter 4. FREEZE-FRAME is designed to give you a way to increase and improve the communication between your heart and mind while reducing stress.

A quick, one-minute exercise, FREEZE-FRAME is invaluable for managing thoughts to prevent the needless depletion of energy. Because this technique increases mental clarity, it will help you make sound decisions, even in what would formerly have been highly stressful situations. Instead of giving way to stress, you'll learn to FREEZE-FRAME—and benefit immediately.

In order to maximize the potential of heart intelligence, it's also important to closely monitor thoughts and feelings. Some of our inner dialogues add energy to our systems, while others deplete us of energy. We'll discuss energy assets and deficits in Chapter 5, before providing an exercise to help you determine how efficiently you're using your available energy. Understanding energy assets and deficits provides a key to accessing your heart intelligence.

Core heart feelings such as appreciation, nonjudgment, and forgiveness increase energy assets and eliminate many deficits. These qualities are like access codes that engage the intelligence of the heart. In the last chapter of this section we'll discuss the "heart power tools"; these utilize core heart feelings to access and apply your heart intelligence.

In Part II you will:

➤ Recognize the importance of eliminating stress

➤ Learn and apply FREEZE-FRAME

➤ Become more aware of your thoughts and feelings and learn how both affect you

➤ Understand the significance of core heart feelings and learn how to apply them to access heart intelligence

# The Risks of Incoherence

Elise was a single mother, divorced just a year, with two young children. She was still feeling the emotional and financial strain of the divorce when her company unexpectedly laid her off. They promised severance pay, but that didn't change the fact that she was now unemployed.

After two weeks of fruitless interviews, Elise became so worried about the future that she couldn't sleep. "How can I pay my bills if I don't get another job soon? What's going to happen to my children? My life's falling apart!" She could feel the stress eating away at her, her thoughts so toxic that they made her predicament worse.

Before long, she was so demoralized that it was hard to muster the confidence to go out on an interview. She was afraid that potential employers could see the hopelessness in her eyes.

Finally, in desperation, she applied for a job she didn't want but was pretty sure she could get. The company had a reputation for treating employees badly and paying peanuts, so she'd saved it as a last resort, figuring that she wouldn't work there unless she had to. It hit her pretty hard when they turned her down.

The night of that rejection, Elise put the kids to bed in a daze and went out to sit on the porch alone. If she couldn't find the money to make her mortgage payment in just a couple of weeks, she'd lose her house. Then her ex-husband might sue for custody. Everything she loved could be taken away. She stared out into the darkness, filled with despair.

Having exhausted every resource she could think of, Elise was left only with herself. She suddenly realized that if *she* didn't pull herself out of this problem, no one would. Oddly enough, the idea encouraged her. As she sat quietly and pulled on every inner resource she had, she began to feel a sense of release—even peace—and an openness to new possibilities. The corporate environment had never really suited her. What if she could open a consulting business and make it on her own? What if this were the chance she'd been waiting for?

Elise didn't know it, but she was tapping into her heart's capacity for hope. Buried under a mountain of fears and outdated expectations, the love and optimism she'd once known had been stifled. But her own natural resilience allowed her to instinctively turn to her heart at that moment of great despair.

And once Elise began to tap into her heart, she found it increasingly easy to imagine new possibilities. Creative ways to start her own business and solve her financial problems began to emerge—not because she had "cheered herself up" but for very clear, scientifically measurable reasons. Aligning herself with her core heart feelings had brought her system out of turmoil and into coherence.

## Internal Coherence

If you're able to make out the words on this page, it's in part because of the light illuminating them. Whether that light is sunlight or artificial light, it's diffuse—that is, spread out—not highly focused. Its particles are dancing around you in seemingly random patterns. They're incoherent, in other words—and it's a good thing they are. If they were focused in a unified pattern, those same light particles would form a brilliant laser beam that would burn a hole in the page and then cut right through the book.

Coherence is more than a powerful, harmonious concept, like everyone humming a tune in unison. It's the state that makes the difference between a book light and a laser beam. Understanding how mental and emotional energy can become coherent, and then putting that understanding into practice, is an essential part of the HeartMath Solution. Inner coherence is a benchmark of intelligence and a cornerstone of effective living. It can be a powerful force in *your* life.

There are high levels of coherent organization and patterning throughout nature. In fact, if our very cells didn't maintain a sense of order and consistency, we'd fall apart. Intuitively, it's easy to grasp that a certain degree of coherence is essential in any living organism.

When a system is coherent, virtually no energy is wasted, because all its components are operating in harmony. It follows, then, that when every system in the body is aligned, your personal power is at its peak.

Most of us have experienced the buoyancy and satisfaction that positive emotional states can create in our lives. At such moments of buoyancy, our effectiveness at big tasks and small improves almost effortlessly. Positive emotional states produce that effect because of the coherence they create within the human system.

Learning to cultivate that rewarding state of coherence enhances our ability to adapt, to flex, and to innovate. It allows us to rapidly get back to a feeling of balance and poise after stressful events and to improve communication, health, and overall well-being. A balanced heart and agile mind create access to innate intelligence and an enhanced capacity for greater internal coherence—the optimal state of being.

## Gaining Access

The challenge we face is to achieve greater levels of internal coherence in an age of increasing chaos, complexity, and *in*coherence. It's no longer enough to be smart. We need a new kind of intelligence that's quicker, more reliable, and more flexible than the linear, step-by-step intelligence we're accustomed to using.

Most people in today's society have the sense that time is speeding up, information and energy are racing, events are happening to and around them at a frenzied pace. As a result, stress is on the rise. New research has found that what creates more stress for people than any other stressor is having to shift concepts, intention, and focus to many different tasks, many times an hour. [1]

Unlike thirty years ago, the average person today is called upon to shift concepts at least seven or eight times an hour. Each interruption by a co-worker, client, or loved one (in person or via e-mail, fax, or phone), for example, demands a concept shift. And many of us more than double that average for concept-shifting: it's not unusual for a person to deal with ten or twenty (or even more) concept shifts in an hour (topping one hundred shifts in a single eight- to ten-hour workday). Given that rapid-fire concept-shifting, it's no wonder that the optimal state of internal coherence is getting harder to maintain—and that stress is on the rise.

Getting our hearts and heads in sync increases the coherence between heart and brain, allowing us to operate at optimal performance levels. [2] But when we're out of sync, our overall awareness is reduced and we diminish the skills we already have. Think of the heart as a radio transmitter broadcasting twenty-four hours a day. The quality of the broadcast is governed by every thought and feeling we have. When our thoughts are fuzzy or chaotic, the broadcast is full of static. We can't receive the whole transmission. Perceptually, we may notice only that we feel irritable or distracted, but that "static" impacts every subsystem of our bodies, clear down to the cellular level.

Lack of coherence affects our vision, listening ability, reaction time, mental clarity, feeling states, and sensitivity. Not only is our overall functioning impaired by incoherence, but that state robs us of a sense of real satisfaction. Even if we do something that we usually find fulfilling, we can feel only a limited portion of that fulfillment when our system is misfiring and out of sync.

Unfortunately, it doesn't take much to create enough static that our perception is impaired. Something as simple as a pointed remark by a friend or relative can make us so angry that we can't think straight. Only later do we think, "What I *should* have said is . . . !" We can't think clearly when we're upset because we're literally incoherent. Our heart rhythms have become disordered and incoherent. This inhibits the higher centers of our brains from working as efficiently as they could. [2] The reason we think of what we should've said *later* is that, after we calm down, our system is functioning more coherently again. We're back in balance, so we can see the situation from a different perspective—our own perspective, free from stress.

It's a vicious circle: stress destroys coherence, and incoherence causes stress. And that's bad news. Stress is much more dangerous than we've thought. Even an occasional stressful experience has a damaging effect on our bodies. We're built with the capacity to tolerate a certain amount of stress. But chronic stress—along with negative attitudes such as hostility, anger, and depression—will sicken and eventually kill us. [3–5] Stress doesn't just pass through us like a fleeting mood. It grips us and doesn't let go, changing our physiology and altering our health.

## The Damaging Effects of Stress

According to the American Institute of Stress, as many as 75 to 90 percent of all visits to primary-care physicians result from stress-related disorders. [6] To cope with these complaints, Americans alone consume five billion tranquilizers, five billion barbiturates, three billion amphetamines, and sixteen thousand *tons* of aspirin (not including ibuprofen and acetaminophen) every year. [7]

Medical science continues to make great strides in connecting external factors such as diet, lifestyle, and environment to our most serious diseases. We now take it for granted that high blood cholesterol, diabetes mellitus, and cigarette smoking are high-risk factors for heart disease. Yet in over *half* of the new cases of heart disease, none of these risk factors is present. [8]

In his 1988 landmark study, Dr. Hans Eysenck of the University of London reported that unmanaged reactions to stress were more predictive of death from cancer and heart disease than cigarette smoking. [9]

In fact, in the aftermath of a heart attack, the greatest predictors of recovery aren't physiological factors—such as an arterial blockage or the condition of the heart itself—but emotional factors. A startling report by the secretary of the federal Department of Health, Education, and Welfare revealed that job satisfaction and "overall happiness" are the factors most likely to determine a patient's recovery. A growing body of compelling scientific evidence demonstrates the direct impact of mental and emotional attitudes on health and well-being:

- In a ten-year study, people who were unable to effectively manage their stress had a 40 percent higher death rate than nonstressed individuals. [9]

- A Harvard Medical School study of 1,623 heart attack survivors found that when subjects got angry during emotional conflicts, their risk of subsequent heart attacks was more than double that of those that remained calm. [10]

- A twenty-year study of over 1,700 older men conducted by the Harvard School of Public Health found that worry about social conditions, health, and personal finances significantly increased the risk of coronary heart disease. [11]

- In one study of 202 professional women, tension between career and personal commitment to spouse, children, and friends was the factor that differentiated those with heart disease from those who were healthy. [12]

- An international study of 2,829 people between the ages of fifty-five and eighty-five found that individuals who reported the highest levels of personal "mastery"—feelings of control over life events—had a nearly 60 percent lower risk of death compared with those who felt relatively helpless in the face of life's challenges. [13]

- According to a Mayo Clinic study of individuals with heart disease, psychological stress was the strongest predictor of future cardiac events, including cardiac death, cardiac arrest, and heart attack. [14]

We hear so many heart disease statistics from newspapers, magazines, health books, and TV that most of us glaze over the issue of heart disease until it affects us personally. A close friend or family member develops heart disease, and then we start wondering how it happened and what can be done about it. Or our doctor warns us that we're at risk ourselves, and suddenly we have an alarmed interest.

What we don't realize is that a heart attack or heart disease happens when something has been going wrong for a long period of time and finally breaks down. The real ailment isn't the final precipitating factor; it's what happened between good health and the disease.

Stress is the ailment to be concerned about. If we live in a stressed-out state all the time, we become used to imbalance. Some of us grew up in homes where anger, depression, or disappointment were common, so we assume that the stress those emotional states cause us is normal. In a metropolitan area, almost everyone around us seems to be rushing, distracted, and hounded by stress—again, it seems normal. No matter where we live, it's easy to find complaining, unhappy people who are quick to notice what's wrong with life instead of finding things to appreciate. But no matter how common this behavior is—how seemingly "normal"—it has serious consequences for our health.

We have two choices: continue to blame the world for our stress, or take responsibility for own reactions and deliberately change our emotional climate. There can no longer be any doubt about it. Most heart problems are the extreme outcome of years of inner stress.

## Chronic Stress

I n 1997 the *Journal of the American Medical Association* published a Duke University study showing that common emotions such as tension, frustration, and sadness can trigger a drop in the blood supply to the heart. In daily life, these emotions more than *double* the risk of myocardial ischemia, an insufficient blood supply to heart tissue that can be a precursor to a heart attack. [15]

According to Dr. Murray Mittleman and Malcolm Maclure at Harvard University, Dr. Gullette's findings in that 1997 study "suggest that prior studies of rare, extremely stressful events, such as earthquakes or war, presented only 'the tip of the iceberg.' By this we refer to the finding that low levels of stress commonly experienced in everyday life can trigger the onset of myocardial ischemia." [16]

Stress is the body and mind's response to any pressure that disrupts their normal balance. It occurs when our perceptions of events don't meet our expectations *and we don't manage our reaction to the disappointment.* Stress—that unmanaged reaction—expresses itself as resistance, tension, strain, or frustration, throwing off our physiological and psychological equilibrium and keeping us out of sync. If our equilibrium is disturbed for long, the stress becomes disabling. We fade from overload, feel emotionally shut down, and eventually get sick.

Today it's recognized that the body's stress response encompasses more than fourteen hundred known physical and chemical reactions and over thirty different hormones and neurotransmitters. The two key physiological systems that coordinate the body's response to stress are the autonomic nervous system, which reacts almost immediately, and the hormonal system, whose reactions occur and persist over a longer time. But even organs that aren't considered part of either of these systems, such as the stomach and kidneys, also pour out hormones to accomplish the body's vast response to stress. [4]

When we experience stress, our bodies quickly react by releasing the hormone adrenaline into the bloodstream. Adrenaline elevates our heart rate and blood pressure, tenses up our muscles, and speeds our breathing, preparing us to confront the threat or run for our lives. Other hormones, including noradrenaline and cortisol, are also activated under stress. If not checked, the perpetual release of these hormones sears the body like acid. Even *hours* after the stress has subsided, these hormonal levels can remain high.

Cortisol has come to be known as the "stress hormone" because of the extensive role it plays in the body's response to stress. In balanced amounts, cortisol is essential for the healthy functioning of our bodies, but when levels rise too high, it can be extremely damaging to our system. When we're under chronic stress and our bodies produce high levels of cortisol over long periods of time, the brain's internal thermostat resets and directs the body to maintain a higher level of cortisol production, thinking that this is normal. Chronically elevated levels of cortisol have been shown to impair immune function [17], reduce glucose utilization [18], increase bone loss and promote osteoporosis [19], reduce muscle mass, inhibit skin growth and regeneration [20], increase fat accumulation (especially around the waist and hips) [21], impair memory and learning, and destroy brain cells. [22, 23]

Chronic stress accumulates day by day, week by week, year by year. For most people, it's the *daily* accumulation that does the most damage; the little stresses add up to far more than the big jolts do. We adjust to everyday stress, but it's a totally unnecessary habit, and the steady biochemical pounding that results takes its toll on our bodies.

We accommodate stress because we don't realize how serious the consequences are and because it's become such a part of the routine that it feels normal to us. After all, aren't all our friends going through the same thing?

We so easily push away feelings of defeat and resentment throughout the day that we hardly notice. When things stifle or annoy us, we all have our favorite ways of reacting. Some people immediately lash out in anger, while others use caustic humor to get some sense of compensation. Some turn to drinking, drugs, or binge eating to stave off feelings of frustration or entrapment. And almost all of us complain on a regular basis—whenever we get together with our friends. Since they have armloads of complaints about their lives as well, it seems like an ordinary, almost sociable, thing to do. But this constant stream of incoherent thoughts and emotions drains our strength like an emotional virus while it reinforces a damaging neural habit in our brains, making it easier for us to feel miserable the next time.

When stress becomes chronic, our bodies don't have time to catch up each day. Even if we pause for a few hours to give ourselves a little break from the onslaught, our body chemistry has been altered as surely as if we'd taken a drug. It can't just snap back into place again. After ten shots of whiskey, no cup of coffee is going to make you sober. You have to wait for the effects to subside—without drinking (or, in this case, stressing out) while you wait!

We all have a stress threshold or crisis point, beyond which we become seriously ill. Under mild pressure, the adrenaline and cortisol bursts brought on by stress can lead to a temporary increase in performance, followed by a healthy fatigue that we eliminate by resting. But with unrelenting adrenaline and cortisol arousal, our performance increasingly falls short of the intended mark. [24] Things start to go dramatically downhill.

## The Morality of Stress

The irony is this: our bodies react to stress in exactly the same way whether or not we have a good reason for being stressed. The body doesn't care whether we're right or wrong. Even when we feel perfectly justified in getting angry—when we tell ourselves that anger is the *healthy* response—we pay for it just the same.

Someone cuts you off in traffic. Not only is it rude, but it causes you to slam on your brakes and pull off to the side, which makes the car behind you do the same thing. As you slump over the steering wheel, you think about the fact that you narrowly escaped a three-car pile-up. That idiot driver actually endangered your life! If *that* doesn't justify anger, what does?

But while you fume and curse, your nervous system is thrown into a state of alarm. Your adrenaline rises as your hormones dutifully respond to the anger you're feeling. Whether you're justified or not, you have to ask yourself, Is it worth it? That driver has gone blissfully on his way, ignorant of the danger he caused, but for the next several hours you're going to be paying for your response in a big way.

As far as your body is concerned, it simply doesn't matter whether your anger is justified or not. No matter *why* you're feeling what you're feeling, the physical consequences are the same.

People regularly experience a whole range of different emotions—from love and hate to joy and sorrow. But as psychologists have told us for decades, feelings aren't right or wrong—they're just feelings. In the physical sense, this is literally true. Our body doesn't make a moral judgment about our feelings; it just responds accordingly.

We're so familiar with our justified stress reactions that we move in and out of stressful, incoherent states without any awareness of their damaging effects. Eventually our sensitivities to feeling get shut down, however, and constant, low-grade anxiety or depression sets in.

In the 1997 Duke University study mentioned above, Dr. Gullette was surprised to find that only a minority of heart patients experienced pain. Even though they were in serious danger of a heart attack, they were completely *unaware* that stress was affecting their hearts. [15] Their awareness of their bodies was so diminished that they couldn't feel what was happening.

Most of us have been taught that repressing our emotions is harmful, and there are abundant research studies to support this. For instance, the tendency to repress emotional distress has now been linked to an increased susceptibility to cancer. [9, 25] Other research has shown that repressing anger puts people at higher risk of developing heart disease. [26]

On the other hand, one of the most commonly held beliefs is that it's healthy to have an angry outburst. This notion derives from an early practice of Sigmund Freud, in which he encouraged patients to let their anger out to promote an emotional clearing. It's perhaps not as well known that Freud later discontinued this practice.

Contrary to what we've been taught, science now tells us that "blowing our top" isn't only harmful to our health, but it may actually be *more* damaging to our system than just fuming over angry feelings. In a study conducted by psychologist Aaron Siegman of the University of Maryland, people who reacted with impulsive outbursts of anger proved to be at higher risk for coronary heart disease than people who kept their anger inside. [27]

For people who have long-standing denial of their emotions, psychology has provided the valuable service of helping them become aware of what they're feeling. However, psychologists are coming to realize that reliving angry or hurtful feelings doesn't make them disappear. Instead, it actually reinforces the emotional pattern in the brain's neural circuitry. This leads to more anger and aggression. Talking about how mad something made you can actually reignite the anger, giving it more power to do your body harm.

Indulging anger is expensive in more ways than one. The federal Department of Transportation reports that road rage and aggressive driving are factors in one-third of traffic accidents involving injury and two-thirds of those resulting in death. [28] Other studies have shown that the inability to control anger figures prominently in lost promotions, firings, and forced retirements. [1]

So if we can't express it or repress it, what do we do when we feel angry? The answer is to recognize the anger but choose to respond to the situation differently. Easier said than done, right? Can you imagine trying to strong-arm your anger into another, more amicable feeling? It would never work. Determination alone doesn't cut it. It takes a new intelligence to understand and manage your emotions. By getting your head and heart in coherence and allowing heart intelligence to work for you, you have a realistic chance of transforming your anger in a healthy way.

## Signals from the Heart

When we look at the brain and heart in light of our new scientific understanding of their powerful inner teamwork, a hopeful picture emerges. Instead of seeing the brain as the sole source of our intelligence, we begin to realize that it's a remarkable partner to our heart, not its master. When properly synchronized, it works in harmony with the heart, tuned in to "the heart's code"—a phrase coined by Dr. Paul Pearsall. [29] It's heart intelligence, working in consort with the head, that gives us the ability to eliminate stress. The best prescription for stress reduction is this: heart + head = coherence.

For years, doctors have been able to see and measure the effects of deep hostility through electrocardiography. [30] A doctor can place electrodes on your earlobes, toes, or anywhere else on your body and record your heartbeat on an electrocardiogram (ECG). Unlike any other internal pulse, the heartbeat is so strong that it can be measured at any point on the body. Its electromagnetic signal permeates every cell.

Recently, scientists have come up with more sophisticated ways to analyze ECG readouts. By applying the techniques of spectral analysis, they've been able to observe that heart rhythms (HRV patterns)—which, as we've seen, are influenced by emotions such as frustration and anger as well as love, care, compassion, and appreciation—affect the frequency patterns in the ECG itself. In other words, *our feelings affect the information contained in the heart's electromagnetic signal.* What spectral analysis has revealed is that when the heart rhythms become more ordered or *coherent,* the electromagnetic field produced by the heart becomes more coherent as well. [31, 32]

Spectral analysis determines what mixture of individual frequencies is contained within an electrical signal. It's like putting a chocolate cake into a machine that gives you a readout specifying how much flour, sugar, eggs, butter, salt, baking powder, and chocolate make up that cake. When it comes to our heart rhythms, spectral analysis shows researchers how coherent our rhythms are. From this information they can also determine the degree of coherence in the heart's electrical broadcast to all our cells and to the people around us.

In one study conducted at the Institute of HeartMath, spectral analysis was applied to the heart rhythm data recorded in someone who was feeling frustrated. Remember the graph in Chapter 2 (Figure 2.4) showing what an incoherent HRV pattern resulting from anger looks like? Now take a look at Figure 3.1. The left-hand side of the figure shows the *frequency spectrum* view of the person's heart rhythms during frustration. This graph illustrates that when we're frustrated, the frequency structure of the heart's rhythmic pattern becomes disordered or incoherent. This indicates disorder in the functioning of the autonomic nervous system. When the heart is operating in this disordered mode, it broadcasts an incoherent electromagnetic signal throughout the body and out into the space around us.

In the same study, scientists monitored the heart rhythms of someone feeling sincere appreciation. (Look back at Figure 2.5 to remember what these coherent heart rhythms look like.) The right-hand panel in Figure 3.1 shows the frequency spectrum of this data. As you can see, the frequency pattern looks very different from that of someone in a state of frustration. This graph illustrates that

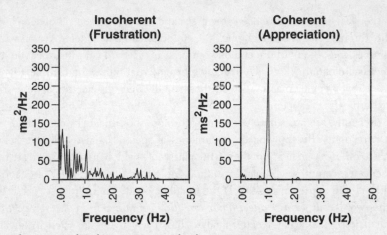

**Incoherent and Coherent Heart Rhythms: Frequency Spectra**

FIGURE 3.1. This figure shows the *frequency spectra* of a person's heart rhythms during different emotional states. These graphs result from the spectral analysis of heart rate variability patterns. Spectral analysis breaks down the overall heart rhythm pattern into the different individual frequencies that make it up. The left-hand graph shows the frequency spectrum of the heart rhythms generated by a person feeling frustration. This is called an *incoherent* spectrum, because the frequencies are scattered and disordered. In this state, there's disorder in the autonomic nervous system and in the electromagnetic field broadcast by the heart. The right-hand graph shows the frequency spectrum of the heart rhythms produced by a person feeling sincere appreciation. This is called a *coherent* spectrum, because the frequency structure of the heart's rhythms is ordered and harmonious. In this state, there's increased harmony in the autonomic nervous system, and the heart's electromagnetic field also becomes more coherent.

when we're feeling appreciation, the two branches of our autonomic nervous work together with increased harmony to produce a single, coherent heart rhythm. When your heart rhythm frequency spectrum looks like the one on the right, you're in a state of *inner entrainment*. In this state of internal balance, the patterns in the electromagnetic field produced by your heart also become more coherent and harmonious. [32]

Remember, this electrical energy radiates information to every cell in and around the body. And your perceptions do affect the signals that are broadcast from your heart, as Figure 3.1 illustrates. The person feeling appreciation generated a coherent wave in that figure, whereas frustration caused the heart's electrical signal to become incoherent. This dramatic difference in internal coherence is caused by a single, very important factor: a difference in perception.

## Overcoming Stress by Changing Perception

The solution to stress management lies in how we perceive the stressors in our lives. It's not really *events* that cause stress; it's how we *perceive* those events. The good news is that since stress is a response—not the event that triggers the response—we can control it.

Once we shift our perception of a situation and see it with heart-focused clarity, our potentially stressful reaction can be reduced or released. The Heart-Math Solution allows us to recognize stress as *an untransformed opportunity for empowerment.* Some problems are hard to see as opportunities for empowerment, yet most perceptions, attitudes, actions, and reactions can be transformed with a generous dose of heart coherence.

In the proceedings of the Seventh International Congress on Stress (1995), Dr. Graham Burrows, president of the International Society for Investigation of Stress, announced that after reviewing years' worth of research on stress, he'd concluded that the problem had been reduced to two basic causes: (1) problems in perception and (2) problems in communication. [33] We can't necessarily change events in life, but we can broaden our perception of them. That's the secret to managing and reducing stress. Improved communication between the heart and the brain follows, and coherence is achieved.

As we come to understand that stress starts with perception, we can observe how each perception starts a cascade of biological effects that color our next perception and reaction—and the next and the next. By paying attention to our perceptions and reactions, then addressing them with heart intelligence, we can eliminate the chronic stress that seeps through our bodies like a slow poison. Learning how to alter our standard stress reactions by perceiving life's events from a place of intuition, balance, poise, and flexibility requires a major shift, though—a shift from head to heart.

The power to think yourself into misery lies within you. But so does the power to stop that process. And which use of power you choose will determine your quality of life. As we've seen, lack of self-management causes a continuous and damaging stress buildup in your system. Much misery—emotional and physical—results when the mind bounces back and forth with anxious thoughts about the day, the future, the past, wondering what it should be doing, second-guessing itself all the time, and dragging old emotions with it. To disperse the stress that accumulates as a result of all this cogitating, the mind looks for stimulating diversions and mindless tasks, rarely seeing that *it* is the cause of the stress—until there's a crash. Then the mind starts to question its approach and looks to the heart for help in picking up the pieces.

It's possible to stop this self-destructive chain of events. By harnessing the power and intelligence of your heart now—and by getting your head and heart in sync—you can reduce (or even eliminate) much of your stress before it takes an unwanted toll, thereby freeing yourself up to make more efficient choices. But reducing stress is a process that has to be undertaken in stages. It's not about perfection but about making steady improvement. Here are four important points to remember about stress:

- Stress is a matter of perception. It isn't events themselves that are stressful; it's our perception of them.

- Stress isn't about just the major problems in life. Stress accumulates as a result of our not managing the little things—our habitual reactions, actions, opinions, irritations, and frustrations.

- Resentment, anger, frustration, worry, disappointment—all negative emotional states, justified or not, take a toll on your heart, your brain, and the rest of your body.

- There's hope. By learning to access your core heart power and the higher-heart feelings associated with it, you can bring your system into increased coherence. This will give you new perceptions and the intelligence you need to transform stress into an opportunity for empowerment.

Accessing the intelligence of the heart—bringing about balance and clarity of perception—is an effective stress-reducing prescription. If you're sincere in your quest for stress management, you can achieve quick results by practicing the next technique in the HeartMath Solution: FREEZE-FRAME.

With practice, you'll learn to cast off habitual negative reactions, grim perspectives, and dissatisfied judgments and begin to live more "from the heart." Although this approach represents a dramatic change in focus for most people, it's not as hard as it sounds. The more you understand the intelligence of the heart, the more power you'll have to shape your perceptions, reduce your stress, increase coherence and creativity, and become the master of your own reality.

## KEY POINTS TO REMEMBER

➤ Positive emotional states create coherence in the human system. Distress creates incoherence.

➤ When a system is coherent, virtually no energy is wasted, because its components are operating in sync.

➤ By learning to access your core heart power and the higher-heart feelings associated with it, you can bring your system into increased coherence.

➤ As you learn to establish balance and harmony between your head and your heart, you'll gain a more intelligent perspective on your stress. By applying new intelligence to stress, you can decrease its power to drain your energy.

➤ Physiologically, it simply doesn't matter whether your anger is justified or not. The body doesn't make moral judgments about feelings; it just responds accordingly.

➤ The real ailment in today's society is what goes on between good health and the manifestation of disease—stress accumulation and decreased quality of life.

➤ Accessing the intelligence of the heart—bringing about balance and clarity of perception—is an effective stress-reducing prescription. It will give you the intelligence you need to transform stress into an opportunity for empowerment.

CHAPTER 4

# FREEZE-FRAME

Before she came to HeartMath, Patricia Chapman was a walking time bomb. Her heart was racing at seven hundred extra beats per hour. Doctors told her the likelihood of sudden death from her condition was high.

"I was trying to be the perfect mother, the perfect wife, the perfect employee," Patricia explained. "I used to sleep four hours a night because there was so much to do. I was so used to that adrenaline rush, I didn't know what it was like not to have it."

Although Patricia had a high-stress job at a global computer company, the pace inside her body was killing her. She took extended sick leave. The doctors had given her beta blockers for arrhythmia as well as Valium after a ventricular tachycardia episode and four surgeries—she almost died from the continued accelerated speed of her heart.

When Patricia came to a HeartMath seminar in the fall of 1995 at the advice of one of her physicians, her hair was falling out, she had stomachaches and headaches all the time, and none of her doctors seemed to be able to do much about it.

Realizing that she was in a life-or-death situation, Patricia was determined to try out HeartMath and practice FREEZE-FRAME on a regular basis. "After my weekend at HeartMath, whenever that adrenaline would start to rush again, I was able to stop the trigger. The first day back to work, I got up eight times and went to the ladies' room, shut myself in, and closed my eyes. That's where I did the FREEZE-FRAME. Now I don't need to close my eyes and I can pull myself back into balance without going anywhere."

Her colleagues immediately noticed a difference—less stress and tension and more ease, even during particularly hectic work periods. Her specialists at Stanford University were particularly impressed.

Within a few weeks, her doctors were able to take her off of Valium; within five months, they decreased the drugs that control her arrhythmia in half; and within nine months, she had a normal twenty-four-hour ECG recording. There have been no further episodes of ventricular tachycardia. Since she made no other medical, lifestyle, dietary, or exercise changes, Patricia attributes these profound improvements to her use of HeartMath Solution tools and techniques.

Over four years later, Patricia is still practicing FREEZE-FRAME regularly. Her heart is beating at a normal rate; the ominous time bomb has stopped ticking. She believes that her practice of this heart-focus technique has given her her life back. "I now feel calm and absolutely incredible," she says.

Patricia's story, like that of many others, makes it clear that the sincere application of heart intelligence can have a dramatic impact on a person's life. Patricia brought about these changes by using FREEZE-FRAME. [1]

## What Is FREEZE-FRAME?

The term "freeze-frame" is movie lingo for stopping a film at a single frame to take a closer look. As you know, a movie is made up of countless frames of film. The projector showing the film runs the sequence of frames past a powerful light so quickly that we perceive them as continuous and unseamed. Together those separate frames create the movement that draws us into the story. If we want to see a still shot of one of the moments flashing by, we have to stop the projector—or *freeze the frame.* [2]

We can look at life as a high-speed movie. We get so caught up in the momentum of the story that it's easy to forget that it's made up of individual moments. From one minute to the next, we have an astonishing range of thoughts, emotions, and experiences that make up our lives.

Think about it. How much has happened inside you since you started reading just this chapter? Maybe the phone rang or you were otherwise interrupted. Maybe you had to move around to get comfortable or find the right lighting. Maybe a certain phrase you read reminded you of something else and your mind began to wander. Each of these events left a mental or emotional trail in your internal world.

If the interruption was enjoyable, you returned to your reading in a pleasant frame of mind. If it wasn't enjoyable, your discomfort was subtly—or not so subtly—woven into your experience as you continued to read. You get the point: each response leads into the next frame. You're writing the story of your life one moment at a time.

The FREEZE-FRAME technique gives you the power to stop your reaction to the movie at any moment. It lets you call a time-out to gain a clearer perspective on what's happening in a single frame. By helping you align your head and your heart, it gives you quick and efficient access to heart intelligence.

Going to your heart through FREEZE-FRAME reduces stress, but it does more than that. It shifts your perspective, allowing you to tap into a deeper source of intuition and power. FREEZE-FRAME uses the power of the heart to help manage the mind. Because our mental, emotional, and physical systems are all interconnected, FREEZE-FRAME also has a powerful effect on our emotions and biology. There are other techniques presented in this book that are designed specifically for managing the emotions and regenerating the body, but FREEZE-FRAME is the quickest, easiest way to engage heart intelligence and bring about a new degree of coherence in all of our systems.

This simple, five-step technique creates a harmonious relationship between the head and the heart. [2] It allows us to edit the next frame in the movie from a point of balance and understanding in order to make smart moves in life. It helps reduce stressful *self-poisoning* and gives us *poise* instead. With practice, we can learn to systematically weave heart intelligence into our daily lives.

When we learn a new physical skill, such as golf, tennis, or dance—or even a dangerous skill such as skydiving—chances are our teacher will remind us to relax and flow with the rhythm of the sport. Good teachers know that when our bodies are free from tension and in harmony—head working with heart—we're able to access more of our natural abilities. The greatest athletes and dancers are those who can relax as they focus on what they're doing. Whenever they achieve that balance between head and heart, their performance visibly improves.

You see it a lot in competitive team sports. Every sports fan is aware that no matter how good his team is, some games are magic. A game like that exceeds everybody's expectations. For whatever reason, the players work together like the components of a well-oiled machine. It looks as if they can read each other's minds. Their individual skills as players are magnified because they're in harmony, in sync with one another.

On the other hand, when a team is out of sync, nothing seems to work right. Pacing on the sidelines, the coach starts to mutter under his breath. He can't believe what he's seeing. Not only is his team losing, they're playing like losers! Everything is off—their timing, their technique, their coordination. Chances are a coach in this position will call a time-out. If he can give his team a break, they can regroup and come back to the game more united.

The coach is also likely to give the team a rousing pep talk. He knows that if they lose heart at a moment like this, all their talent, skill, and practice will go to waste. The same is true for you. From time to time it's a good strategic move to call a time-out and regroup your internal team—your head and your heart.

You may think you don't have time to take a break, but you do: FREEZE-FRAME was designed to work quickly. The brief mental time-out it gives you allows you to gain access—on the spot—to the balancing power of the heart and the revitalizing insights of heart intelligence.

## The Five Steps of FREEZE-FRAME

Here are the five steps of the Freeze-Frame technique:

1. Recognize the stressful feeling and FREEZE-FRAME it! Take a time-out.
2. Make a sincere effort to shift your focus away from the racing mind or disturbed emotions to the area around your heart. Pretend you're breathing through your heart to help focus your energy in this area. Keep your focus there for ten seconds or more.
3. Recall a positive, fun feeling or time you've had in life and try to re-experience it.
4. Now, using your intuition, common sense, and sincerity, ask your heart, What would be a more efficient response to the situation, one that would minimize future stress?
5. Listen to what your heart says in answer to your question. (It's an effective way to put your reactive mind and emotions in check and an in-house source of commonsense solutions!)

FREEZE-FRAME isn't hard to learn. With practice, this technique becomes almost second nature. But don't let its simplicity fool you. Simplicity is efficient, and it usually manifests when complexity has finally been unraveled. Systematic practice of these five steps will yield substantial results. FREEZE-FRAME provides a doorway to intuitive intelligence and builds a reliable bridge between heart and head. Before you try the technique, let's further explain each of the steps.

## Step 1

*Recognize the stressful feeling and* FREEZE-FRAME *it! Take a time-out.*

Anytime we feel out of balance mentally or emotionally, we experience a certain degree of stress. Yet because we've adapted to an undercurrent of stress in our lives, we often don't recognize it even when it's eating away at us. As the momentum of daily activity slowly builds, we experience one little stress response after another. Before we know it, we're operating at less than maximum capacity. Yet only by becoming aware of when we're in stress do we have the chance to stop stress.

As we described in Chapter 3, we first experience stress mentally and emotionally through our perceptions. Our bodies generally give us some signals when we're experiencing too much stress. We may develop tension in our muscles; perhaps our shoulders and neck get tight. We may find that our stomach gets queasy or our head starts to ache or we feel edgy. If our stress is left unchecked, we can become confused and forget where we were going or what we were doing. Then it's all that much easier to be abrupt with people and take everything personally. In any case, we go to bed exhausted. The early-warning signs of stress differ in each one of us. The important thing is that we learn to recognize our own cues for stress.

Once we've noticed the stress—at that very moment—we must pause and take a time-out, acknowledging that we need a new perspective and stepping back from the problem. This can be challenging, because we get so caught up in responsibilities and activities.

This first step of FREEZE-FRAME is like pushing the pause button on a VCR to stop a movie. In this case, though, it's the movie of our lives. Think about it this way: if we want to be the director of our own movie—exert some control over the action—we have to stop being just one of the characters and step back to see the whole picture.

## Step 2

*Make a sincere effort to shift your focus away from the racing mind or disturbed emotions to the area around your heart. Pretend you're breathing through your heart to help focus your energy in this area. Keep your focus there for ten seconds or more.*

By shifting focus away from the problem and toward the heart, we transfer energy from our perception of the problem to possibilities for its solution.

Focusing in the area of the heart might seem like just a convenient way to distract the mind. While it's true that this step helps pull mental focus away from the problem, there's more to it than that. Shifting focus from head to heart improves nervous system balance, heightens cardiovascular efficiency, and enhances communication between heart and brain, bringing more coherence to the mind and emotions. [3–6]

If you have difficulty shifting your attention to the area around the heart, try this: focus on your left big toe; wiggle it, see how it feels, and notice how easy it is to redirect your attention to this area. Now try shifting your attention to the area around your heart. Pretend that your breath is going in and out through the area of the heart (or hold your hand over your heart) to help focus your attention in this area. Keep your focus there for ten seconds or more.

## Step 3

*Recall a positive, fun feeling or time you've had in life and try to reexperience it.*

You might, for example, recall a relaxing vacation; the love you feel for a child, spouse, or parent; a special moment you spent in nature; the appreciation you feel for someone or something in your life. Remember the *feeling* you had, such as joy, appreciation, care, compassion, or love. In the lab, it's been shown that experiencing these core heart feelings is what provides regeneration to the nervous system, the immune system, and the hormonal system, facilitating health and well-being. [3, 6–8] And these positive feelings also assist us in seeing the world with more clarity, discernment, and balance.

What's important in this step is to reexperience the *feeling*. This isn't just mental visualization—picturing something in our minds. For instance, someone who uses her last vacation in Hawaii to trigger a positive feeling may remember the moonlight shining on the water or the wind gently blowing through the palm trees as she stood with her husband on the beach. But the question is, What did that experience *feel* like, not (or not *just*), What did it *look* like? This step is intended to evoke the feeling memory.

We've trained tens of thousands of people in FREEZE-FRAME, and for many of them this third step has been the most difficult. For people who are shut off from the heart, recalling a positive feeling can be hard. And it's harder still when the present situation is extremely stressful and emotionally charged. If you have trouble accessing positive feelings on demand, simply do the best you can. Just the effort of shifting your focus to a feeling such as appreciation, whether from the past or in the present, will help you neutralize the negative reaction.

Dr. Richard Podell, an internist and clinical professor in family medicine at the University of Medicine and Dentistry of New Jersey—and a certified FREEZE-FRAME trainer—has used and taught FREEZE-FRAME for about three years. Dr. Podell has trained over one hundred patients, who typically master the technique in two one-hour sessions. He's discovered that once a patient has identified the image, experience, or person that best triggers feelings of appreciation, care, or love, the process becomes clear and results are significant.

With a little effort, people can find key triggers that activate the positive heart feelings needed in this step. Dr. Bruce Wilson, a cardiologist who includes FREEZE-FRAME as a formal component in the cardiac rehabilitation program at his hospital in Milwaukee, Wisconsin, shares the experience of one of the many patients to whom he's taught FREEZE-FRAME: "When I was in Vietnam," the patient said, "we were lying in the trenches, scared all the time. We thought we were going to die every day. But there was this one morning in particular when the sun came up—brilliant orange—and I could see through the trees. And just for a second, I was so glad to be alive. When I do a FREEZE-FRAME, I remember that wonderful, relaxed feeling. That's what comes to me every time."

## Step 4

*Now, using your intuition, common sense, and sincerity, ask your heart, What would be a more efficient response to the situation, one that would minimize future stress?*

In this step, still keeping your focus in the area around your heart, simply ask, What would be a more efficient response to the situation—one that would minimize future stress? By asking this question from the heart, your intuition, common sense, and sincerity will become more active and available. While you won't necessarily have crystal-clear insights every time you ask, you'll gradually increase your capacity to arrive at convenient and practical solutions.

As you practice this step, remember to stay focused in the area around the heart. This helps keep you anchored so that you don't jump right back into the head.

## Step 5

*Listen to what your heart says in answer to your question. (It's an effective way to put your reactive mind and emotions in check and an in-house source of common-sense solutions!)*

Once the noise of your mind and emotions is quieted, you can hear what some call the "still, small voice." Finding this inner wisdom or intuition requires making the shift from head to heart—a shift that the previous four steps will have helped you to make. Now that you're heart-focused, try to be still inside; relax and casually listen for a signal from the heart. As your system becomes more coherent, the brain waves will begin to synchronize with the heart rhythms [3], which will facilitate cortical function (discussed in Chapter 2) and provide increased access to potential intelligence. This process results in a shift in perception and access to new information.

Sometimes the answers we arrive at through FREEZE-FRAME seem very simple; in fact, sometimes they're merely verification of something we already knew. Other times, though, we experience a download of new information and fresh perspectives. Still other times we may get a feeling rather than a clear answer. As we listen to our heart signals, more often than not we'll experience some type of shift in energy or perception. What's important here is that we make an effort to follow the best heart directive we can, even if it's a fleeting feeling (or worse, something we don't *want* to hear, such as, "Let it go and move on").

Bill, an entrepreneur who'd had quadruple bypass surgery and aorta replacement, had a hard time connecting with his heart. But when he read about the effects that FREEZE-FRAME could have on the heart, he decided to give it a try. The first thing he used the technique on was his road rage. Because he traveled every day for work, he had a lot of opportunities to put it to use. Before long, his outrage at other drivers had been transformed by FREEZE-FRAME; he soon found that he was only rarely getting angry, and even then only mildly. So he decided to try FREEZE-FRAME on other issues.

It was no secret to Bill that he hadn't been a pleasure to be around for years. He'd let his frustration with his marriage set the tenor of his life. Somewhere along the way, his relationship with his forty-four-year-old daughter had deteriorated as well.

"I decided to FREEZE-FRAME about my relationship with my daughter one morning while I was driving to work. After going through the steps just that once, I knew I'd changed." Although he didn't have any particular thoughts or insights about the relationship, he was able to let go of his old, rigid mind-set and get in touch with his compassion and love for her again. And that was enough to change everything.

"Now my daughter and I get along fine," he says. "We talk on the phone almost every day, and she says she likes the person I am now. What a rewarding experience!"

# The Biology of FREEZE-FRAME

W hat takes place in our bodies when we FREEZE-FRAME? Whether anything feels different or not, when we sincerely FREEZE-FRAME there's a
greater level of harmony in our heart rhythms. Our nervous system, which regulates heart rate, blood pressure, and many other glands and organs, comes into
increased balance. [3] This allows the perceptual centers of the brain to process
information more efficiently, giving us better access to important information
we already have stored in the brain and allowing new intuitive solutions accessed by the heart and core heart feelings to reach the conscious mind.

As we saw in Chapter 2, this technique has such a balancing effect on heart
rhythms—the strongest rhythms in the body—that the heart pulls many of the
body's other rhythmic biological systems into entrainment, and in that state
they work together more efficiently. As in the earlier sports analogy, our inner
team is now working in harmony.

Figure 4.1 shows how three important rhythmic biological systems interact
before and after FREEZE-FRAME. The test subject whose results are shown was
monitored for ten minutes to assess heart rate variability, pulse transit time (a
measurement of blood pressure), and respiration.

Five minutes (or three hundred seconds) into the experiment, the subject
began to FREEZE-FRAME. The vertical line in the middle of the three-part
graph marks that moment. As you can see, the patterns immediately shifted
from jagged and irregular to ordered and coherent, and all three systems became entrained. His respiration, blood pressure, and nervous system started
working together more efficiently as soon as he engaged his heart. This finding
helps to explain why people like Bill feel in sync without having any way to explain it.

An interesting study on the effects that different emotions have on the autonomic nervous system and the heart, conducted at the Institute by research director Rollin McCraty and his team of scientists, was published in the *American
Journal of Cardiology* in 1995. In this study, FREEZE-FRAME was used as the
method by which research subjects intentionally shifted emotional states in the
moment through heart focus. The results, according to the journal, confirm that
FREEZE-FRAME offers people a new method for improving health and well-
being: "The positive shifts in autonomic nervous system balance that all subjects
were able to achieve in this study through using FREEZE-FRAME may be beneficial in the control of hypertension and in reducing the likelihood of sudden
death in patients with congestive heart failure and coronary artery disease." [3]

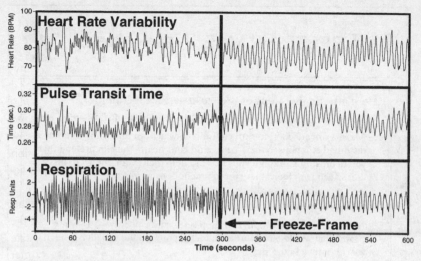

*Entrainment During FREEZE-FRAME*

FIGURE 4.1. This graph shows a person's heart rate variability, pulse transit time, and respiration pattern over ten minutes. At three hundred seconds, the individual FREEZE-FRAMED and all three physiological systems came into entrainment. When our systems are synchronized in this way, they function with increased efficiency, saving valuable energy and promoting health.

## FREEZE-FRAME Exercise

It's now time to have your own experience with FREEZE-FRAME. This is your first attempt, so be careful not to fall prey to unrealistic expectations. It can take several practices before you feel anything or gain any clarity. So don't feel that you're doing something wrong or suspect that you're the only one who "doesn't get it" the first time or two. Listening to your heart isn't hard, but *attuning* to its inner signals is different for everyone and often takes a little practice. Just take it slow and easy and get the fundamentals down. FREEZE-FRAME is a *learned skill* that develops your emotional and heart intelligence as you use it.

Turn now to the FREEZE-FRAME worksheet on page 74 and start with this written exercise. Writing will help you clarify your self-awareness and see links between thoughts, feelings, reactions, and choices. The FREEZE-FRAME worksheet is like the training wheels on a child's first bike. Once you get the hang of this technique, you'll be able to FREEZE-FRAME and connect with your heart power and intuition without having to write everything down.

# FREEZE-FRAME Worksheet

**Here are the five steps of the FREEZE-FRAME technique:**

1. Recognize the stressful feeling, and FREEZE-FRAME it. *Take a time-out!*

2. Make a sincere effort to shift your focus away from the racing mind or disturbed emotions to the area around your heart. You can pretend that you're breathing through your heart to help focus your energy in this area. Keep your focus there for ten seconds or more.

3. Recall a positive, fun feeling or time you've had in life and attempt to re-experience it.

4. Now, using your intuition, common sense and sincerity — ask your heart, what would be a more efficient response to the situation, one that will minimize future stress?

5. Listen to what your heart says in answer to your question. It's an effective way to put your reactive mind and emotions in check — and an "in-house" source of common sense solutions!

**Situation** _____

_____

**Head Reaction** _____

_____

_____

_____

*FREEZE-FRAME*

**Heart intuition response** _____

_____

_____

_____

_____

In doing the FREEZE-FRAME exercise, I shifted from _____ to _____.

1. First, think of a current stressful situation in your life and describe it in a few words under "Situation." *Don't* start with the biggest, most emotionally charged issue you have. If you were going to the gym to work out for the first time, you wouldn't pick up the heaviest weights in the building, would you? Some situations take more muscle than others. Start with a "beginner-level" stress to test your strength, and you can build from there.

2. Under "Head Reaction," write down what you've been going through around this situation: thoughts that keep recurring, feelings and reactions that keep surfacing—whether anger, frustration, worry, impatience, burnout. Please note that the term "head reaction" refers to a combination of thoughts and emotions *generated by the head*, not core heart feelings.

3. After describing the situation and your head reaction, take a minute to review the five steps of FREEZE-FRAME. Then relax and go through each step one at a time. Close your eyes if you like. (While you're learning, closing your eyes makes it easier to shift perception. Once you get the knack of it, though, you can FREEZE-FRAME with eyes open or closed.) When you're ready—having focused in the area of the heart, activated a core heart feeling, and asked your question from the heart— write down what your heart tells you under "Heart Intuition Response."

4. Now review your FREEZE-FRAME worksheet. Read what you wrote under "Head Reaction" and then what you wrote under "Heart Intuition Response." Is there a difference? If so, describe the difference.

5. Now find one or two words that capture the essence of the head reaction—such as "angry," "emotional," or "impatient." Then find one or two words that describe the intuitive perspective— such as "calm," "logical," or "caring." Write those words in the blanks provided on the worksheet. (For example, someone might FREEZE-FRAME a situation and shift from "confusion" to "clarity" or from "anger" to "acceptance.")

Don't worry if you didn't have any life-changing insights. It's important to recognize that you're on a learning curve. Just making the sincere effort to try FREEZE-FRAME is an important step forward. Your skills will improve with practice.

Initially, though, you'll at least feel more balanced and calm. You may even experience a subtle but important attitude or perspective shift. Even if you don't have all the answers you need to resolve your situation, you'll feel clearer about the issue and know that you're headed in the right direction. (Sometimes when people don't get immediate answers, the answer catches up with them later!)

With each repetition, you'll learn to tap more deeply into your heart. As you build up your heart power and improve your FREEZE-FRAME skills, the insights you gain and the shifts in attitude and perspective will come faster and be more profound. Practice is the key.

## What's Different About FREEZE-FRAME?

You may find that your experience while doing the FREEZE-FRAME exercise is similar (at least at first) to things you've felt before. As we said in the beginning, all of us have had the experience of consulting our heart intelligence. So it's natural that the feeling might seem familiar.

One of the great advantages of the HeartMath Solution is that it allows you to reevoke these states *at will*. Once you have the tools, you can return to your heart systematically, which allows you to cultivate an ever-growing heart intelligence.

But people often ask us, "How is FREEZE-FRAME different from breathing exercises or meditation?" Good question.

For most of us under stress today, our grandparents' advice to stop, take a few deep breaths, and count to ten doesn't bring lasting relief anymore. The mind and emotions start churning again soon after we're done counting. We need something more.

Simply taking a few deep breaths *can* be helpful. This is because our breathing patterns modulate our heart rhythms. In fact, it's possible to entrain our breathing pattern and heart rhythms (without focusing in the area of the heart) through "cognitive" breathing exercises—that is, exercises through which we become aware of how fast and deeply we're breathing and then consciously control our breath rate—if we breathe at the right rate or frequency. [6]

Cognitive breathing exercises *impose* a breathing rhythm on our heart rhythms when we breathe at a slow, rhythmic rate (say, five seconds in and then five seconds out), and that facilitates entrainment. But we've discovered that people find it very difficult to consciously maintain a slow breath rate for very long. It feels a bit uncomfortable, and people quickly tire of breathing this way.

When people focus in the heart and breathe "through" the heart in a relaxed way, smooth, entrained HRV patterns occur more naturally. As a result, they're easier to sustain for longer periods of time. This is because the *heart is the primary regulator* of respiratory rhythm. [9]

FREEZE-FRAME allows a spontaneous entrainment or coherence to naturally emerge, thus bypassing any need for cognitive control of breathing. The mind gets out of the way instead of driving the breathing process. This not only feels good but is easy to sustain.

FREEZE-FRAME also creates a mood shift to harmonious feeling states such as care and appreciation, which helps to create and sustain entrainment between heart and brain. [4] The breathing rate synchronizes to the signals flowing up the nerves from the heart to the brain. [9]

The key to the success of FREEZE-FRAME lies in using the power of your heart to entrain your biological, mental, and emotional systems. You achieve the best results from FREEZE-FRAME when you focus in the area of the heart; take a few slow, full breaths; sincerely feel emotions such as love, care, or appreciation; and then forget about breathing while maintaining that feeling state. With this process, you get the benefit of both slow breathing and the emotional shift of FREEZE-FRAME as you produce and sustain beneficial HRV patterns.

Many meditation and visualization techniques focus in the head—the center of the forehead or the crown—and attempt to use the mind to quiet the mind. Such techniques can be very difficult to master. While researchers see changes in brain waves and other bodily responses (including some reduction in autonomic activity) from meditative states, they rarely see coherence in the heart rhythms.

Even meditation techniques that have you focus in the heart often use only the mind to direct the energy, rather than engaging the core heart feelings needed to let the heart distribute the energy flow. Engaging a core heart feeling shifts heart rhythms into increased coherence—a valuable outcome. Research conducted by the Institute has found that it takes coherence in the heart rhythms to really calm the mind and achieve an intuitive state.

This understanding is what led me (Doc) to develop the FREEZE-FRAME technique in the first place. I found, from my own experience with meditation and prayer practices over twenty years (and from observation of others who used similar practices), that people need long periods of practice and discipline to quiet the mind enough to get the physiological and intuitive benefits of meditation. Even longtime meditators get only limited benefits unless the heart is deeply engaged, so they're often frustrated with their progress.

I deeply respect all the efforts people make and the disciplines they use for going within—their private ways of praying or meditating. In developing

FREEZE-FRAME, I wanted to help people who have no inclination or time to meditate. I also wanted to help those who use prayer, meditation, or other personal growth methods find that deeper place in the heart so that they could gain maximum benefit from their efforts.

Like prayer, FREEZE-FRAME can be done while a person is on the road, waiting for a meeting, riding the bus; it can be done anytime and anywhere. Like meditation, FREEZE-FRAME can be done for longer lengths of time if we choose. However, most people don't have much time, so it's a good tool to use to get quick results.

One of the things people like most about FREEZE-FRAME is that it can be done in the moment—whenever they want deeper peace or need quick intuitive access. It can be achieved in less than a minute, once you're practiced at it. You don't have to go off somewhere alone to meditate. Even if meditation works for you, you can't always escape to a quiet place and spend twenty minutes on your own. When you're in a frustrating meeting at the office or driving screaming kids home from school—your stress level climbing—retreating into an altered state just isn't an option.

The importance of being able to FREEZE-FRAME in *real time*—at the very moment you're under stress—and find inner peace and harmony can't be overemphasized. This immediacy neutralizes the physiological and psychological impacts of stress, frustration, and anxiety *at once*. It cuts off the drain on your nervous, hormonal, and immune systems that would have occurred if you'd allowed the stress response to run its course. When you pause to FREEZE-FRAME and truly engage your heart, you get right back into balance, stopping stress in its tracks. That's why FREEZE-FRAME was designed as a tool to be used *on the spot*.

Any meditation, visualization, prayer, affirmation, or stress-reduction technique can be enhanced by adding focused heart to the process. Jack, a longtime meditator, told us, "I found that after over ten years of daily meditation, FREEZE-FRAME really shifted things for me. I was able to achieve in just a few practices what I'd been trying to find all those years—the ability to feel my heart more deeply and the ability to regain my inner peace more quickly when I lost it. It's especially useful in the midst of daily activity, because that's where I'm most at risk mentally and emotionally."

Whatever techniques you practice, realize that the message of the heart becomes clearer when the mind is quiet. And in order to truly quiet the mind, we need to bring the head into alignment with the heart. The *degree of heart* you put into any health practice—whether diet, exercise, prayer, meditation, or self-help discipline—will be the degree of its effectiveness. FREEZE-FRAME, with its scientifically researched, user-friendly steps, can add coherent heart power to whatever techniques you use.

The HeartMath tools and techniques are designed to be facilitators, not competitors, of personal or spiritual growth methods. We honor any process that helps people find peace, inspiration, well-being, or improved health. FREEZE-FRAME is a convenient, approachable, and efficient way to experience clarity, inner security, and peace whenever you need it.

## Finding the Neutral Zone

B ut let's face it, accessing a positive feeling such as compassion (let alone appreciation) can be difficult at times, especially if the situation is extremely stressful and emotionally charged. In such cases, making the effort to at least become more neutral might be the best we can do. If we can accomplish that, it may be more of a success than we realize.

Don't underestimate the power of the neutral state. It saves energy and provides fertile ground for new insights to grow. The ability to find neutral, and stay put there until the heart clearly reveals what to do, is a sign of balance and maturity. Impulse control—that is, the ability to delay gratification of impulses—is a measure of emotional intelligence. When we manage to reach a neutral state, our heart rhythms soon restore their balance so that we can perceive new options for action, instead of mechanically reacting on impulse and paying for it (and probably regretting it) later.

Thoughts and feelings play a major role in everything we do. It's through these inner processes that we experience our happiness and peace of mind—as well as those terrible days we'd like to forget. FREEZE-FRAME isn't going to change every unpleasant situation we face. Life will still be life. But this technique can help us shift into neutral so that we aren't drained and depleted time after time.

When we're in neutral, we adapt more quickly even if things don't go the way we'd like. Instead of wasting energy judging a person or situation unfavorably, we step back and wait until we can find a deeper level of insight. We don't press forward or back; we hang loose in neutral. And FREEZE-FRAME can get us there. It clears the fog from the window of our mind so that we can see clearly. Then we have the option to reframe what's going on. [2]

The neutral zone is a conduit for objectivity in the moment. Trying to stay neutral while the head is frantically forming opinions and making high-speed judgments is a real challenge. The head wants to come to a conclusion *now*. It longs to say, "I *know* what's happening here!"—whether its opinions are based on reliable information or not.

In every situation that triggers stress, we can hear the racket in our heads and feel the old familiar pull; but if we just keep practicing the first two steps of FREEZE-FRAME, we'll find that neutral point. From there we can ask ourselves, "What if there's more to this situation than I've perceived? What if there's something else I don't know?" It's amazing how much energy is saved in neutral, where we don't automatically let our minds assume that something is one way or the other.

Parents know that it takes a lot of effort to calm down kids who are throwing a temper tantrum, to bring them back into control; but the effort is worthwhile because we love them. Our inner temper tantrums are just as challenging. We all have them at times, and they don't go away on command. Yet the effort to control them is worth it. Try not to be impatient. Have some compassion for yourself, just as you would for your children. Each time you make an effort to FREEZE-FRAME in the heart and find the neutral zone in a stressful situation, you build that muscle a little more. And each time the process gets a little easier.

I (Howard) have a personal FREEZE-FRAME classic about the power of staying in neutral. One day I was flying down to Los Angeles on a business trip and ended up in one of those seats that directly face another row. I had the aisle seat, a young woman sat next to me, and a well-dressed businessman occupied the window seat. Across from us was a young mother with two children—a boy about three years old and a small baby.

Things went fine for a while, but eventually the little boy got restless and started throwing his toy cars all over the place. His mother could see that the car-throwing was irritating the businessman, so she pulled out the boy's tray table and gave him some cookies and a little box of grape juice with a straw in it. Before long the boy was pounding the juice box up and down on the tray table. You guessed it: the container popped out of his hand and flew toward the businessman, spattering him from head to toe with grape juice.

As the mother did her best to appease the man and calm the wiggling child, the baby started crying. The mother, deciding that it was time for a diaper change, pulled off the loaded diaper and set it on the baby's tray table—right in front of me. The entire area was filled with the pungent odor.

As the new diaper was being fastened, the captain came on the intercom to announce that we'd be starting our descent soon. The young woman next to me tapped my arm and said, "Pardon me, sir, but I'm a white-knuckle flyer. Would you mind if I held onto you while we land?"

"Sure," I said, not knowing what to expect. Permission granted, the woman grabbed my forearm with both her hands and dug her head deep into my shoulder.

So there I was, trapped in an airplane with an irate businessman in a grape suit, a terrified woman, a harried young mother, an uncontrollable toddler, a crying baby—and yes, that well-used diaper still staring me in the face.

This seemed like a good time to test the effectiveness of FREEZE-FRAME. I went through the first three steps, but all I could do was find neutral. I had to rest there for awhile, my eyes closed. Then I asked the question, What would be a more efficient way to deal with this situation—one that would minimize future stress?

The first response I got from the heart was to have compassion for everyone involved. It was just plain hard for everybody.

Next I was struck by the humor of it all. I truly did feel compassion for all concerned, but the whole thing suddenly seemed funny to me. I had to open my eyes just to control my laughter, as well as to check the blood supply in my arm. The plane was landing, and the woman's grip had gone to maximum power.

After leaving the plane, I was glad the flight was over—but I had a smile on my face.

## Enhancing Daily Life

We've all had experiences that we wish we could go back and change. Even assuming that we couldn't prevent a difficult situation from happening, we'd like to change the way we handled it, rephrase what we said. Since that's never an option, we need to get things right the first time. The power to stop a rambling mind and settle disturbed emotions so that we can evaluate a stressful situation is inherent in the heart of each person. When we use that power, consciously acting from a point of heart balance, we lessen our need for regret because we connect more naturally with what our *real* self—not our reactive self—wants to think or do.

The first time Rosemary used FREEZE-FRAME was during a week of conflict with her husband and daughter. For her, as for many families, parenting issues were among the most emotionally charged.

"We'd recently learned that our daughter had become sexually active," Rosemary explained. "Scott and I immediately went into stress about it. After several days Scott got into blaming me, and I reacted defensively for myself and protectively for my daughter. I thought he'd turned into a schizophrenic. A personality emerged from him that I didn't know or like.

"When I shared what was happening with one of my dearest friends, she suggested that I try accessing my heart by shifting my awareness to the heart area and breathing through the heart. She took me through the steps of Freeze-Frame, although I didn't know then that that's what it's called. The process seemed very natural.

"During the next interaction with my husband that evening over our daughter, I started reacting in the same old pattern. Then I remembered to try being in my heart by using the steps my friend had taught me. I went through the steps as my husband was talking.

"I sensed a shift immediately. For the first time I was able to hear his fear, his pain, his unresolved issues around his own sexuality and the double standard he had for his sons and daughters. I felt compassion instead of anger and was able to respond from my heart instead of react from my head.

"The energy shift was so powerful that I was almost stunned. Our conflicts resolved very quickly and much more tenderly after that. I was amazed that the power of the heart could give me that much insight."

Freeze-Frame is a valuable tool as we wrestle with personal relationships, but it's also useful in the workplace. Business clients have told us hundreds of stories about how Freeze-Frame has helped them save time and energy. Many have used Freeze-Frame to sort through, prioritize, and weed out the flood of incoming information they face each day. This tool has been especially useful for intact teams—those for whom staying focused on goals, communication, creativity, and team synergy is essential for success.

Dan, a mid-level manager, remarked that meetings were generally the most stressful and draining part of his day. "My job often requires me to be in three or four meetings a day, usually with co-workers I know well," he told us. "One of our managers, Mary, is well known for dragging her points out and repeating things endlessly. It bothers a lot of people, but it hits me especially hard, because I'm pretty concise and don't have much patience. A few days after learning Freeze-Frame, I was listening to Mary in a meeting, feeling my impatience growing, when I suddenly thought of Freeze-Frame. I dropped down into my heart the best I could, and all my judgments left me. I actually felt real compassion for the woman and her need to elaborate on everything. It was wonderfully freeing to be able to listen to her with compassion. It made a difference to the rest of my day and evening."

## Practicing Freeze-Frame

With any new skill, there are potential pitfalls. Forgetting. Feeling discouraged. Not having enough time. Whether you're a businessperson, truck driver, teacher, parent, or student, it's easy to get entangled in the daily routine of life. Changing your routine requires sincere, self-initiated effort.

You can't expect miracles overnight in areas that have been tough for you for years. But you'll be surprised at the progress you can make. Once you begin to see results, that provides motivation to keep going for more heart contact. And as you keep going, it gets smoother and easier, as with any skill. Before long, your common sense and enjoyment of your own heart intelligence will help you remember the technique.

For the next couple of weeks, apply Freeze-Frame to at least four or five situations every day. Here are some helpful suggestions (and you can add your own ideas in the space provided):

*When to Apply Freeze-Frame at Home*

- At transition points (home to work or work to home), so that you leave work at work, leave family conflicts at home, and are fully present in the moment
- Before conversations or phone calls, to enhance sincerity, depth of connection, and listening ability
- Any time communication begins to go off track
- When children are upset, arguing, or acting up
- At the beginning of the day, to set the tone for positive activity, calibrate your system for a coherent day, and clear out the mental and emotional cobwebs from the day or night before
- At the end of the day, to feel positive completion of the day and ensure a good sleep
- Other_____

_____

*When to Apply* Freeze-Frame *at Work*

- At transition points, to renew freshness and coherence (traveling from home to work, work to home; and before and at the end of meetings, procedures, appointments, and phone calls)
- At planning sessions and during other creative ventures
- Before delivering a talk or participating in any event that requires clarity, balance, and maximum intelligence
- After a difficult interaction with a co-worker or client, or before an interaction that may be difficult
- As part of any break—coffee, lunch, evening, weekends, vacation—to add to the refreshment and rejuvenation
- At any stress point or choice point
- Other_____

_____

*Using* Freeze Frame *for Health and Creativity*

- To help with health challenges such as high blood pressure, arrhythmia, tension headaches, PMS, panic attacks, chronic fatigue syndrome, and so on
- To help determine a balanced diet and exercise program
- To encourage creative inspiration
- To improve performance in golf, tennis, or any other sport
- To enhance creative projects such as writing, painting, and hobbies
- Other_____

_____

## Practice Tips

It's helpful to set up a system of simple Freeze-Frame reminders. You can leave yourself notes on the bathroom mirror or on the refrigerator door. You can set your digital watch to beep as a reminder to Freeze-Frame at a particular time. If you work at a computer, you can write a note to yourself on your screensaver to encourage and remind you to practice. You can fill out a

FREEZE-FRAME worksheet to get your heart's intuitive insights on how best to integrate FREEZE-FRAME into your life.

Keep in mind how important it is to FREEZE-FRAME the small stuff. If you wait until a crisis comes up, you may not have enough heart power built up to get the insight you need. Start small and go step by step. Begin with daily irritations, frustrations, and disappointments as they happen, knowing that you're building reserves for bigger, unexpected events later.

One thing is certain: you'll have plenty of chances to practice FREEZE-FRAME. Life is full of potentially stressful situations. If you try using FREEZE-FRAME in these situations as they occur, you'll start to offset the stress. Not only will this put you in a better mood throughout the day, but your body will thank you for it.

You won't have to FREEZE-FRAME for the rest of your life, though. The whole purpose of this one-minute technique is to take you consciously toward an automatic process. Over time, a big change will take place. Instead of having to FREEZE-FRAME at regular intervals or "apply" the technique to stress like antiseptic on a wound, you'll find that you'll stay in the heart and in the flow for longer and longer periods of time.

After awhile, a polarity shift will take place from head to heart. Once you've made that shift, you'll find it uncomfortable *not* to be connected to your heart. On those rare occasions when you react with your head alone, it won't feel right or natural and you'll want to FREEZE-FRAME as a way to quickly reconnect.

Remember that this technique isn't about perfection but about ratios, about upping the percentage of time you stay in rapport with the heart. As you raise that percentage, you increase the flow of appreciative, compassionate, and caring feelings that wash over you all day. Love, instead of stress, becomes your new mode of being.

## KEY POINTS TO REMEMBER

➤ FREEZE-FRAME enhances your power to stop your reaction to the movie of life at any moment. It lets you get a clearer perspective on what's happening in a single frame and allows you to edit the next frame from a point of balance and understanding.

➤ The key to the success of FREEZE-FRAME lies in using the power of your heart to entrain your biological systems. As your brain begins to synchronize with your heart, cortical facilitation can occur. This results in access to new information and a shift in perception.

➤ By shifting focus toward your heart and away from whatever problem you face, you divert energy from your perception of the problem. When you consciously act from a point of heart balance, you connect more naturally with what your real self—not your reactive self—wants to think or do.

➤ Listening to your heart isn't hard, but *attuning* to its inner signals is different for everyone and often takes a little practice.

➤ FREEZE-FRAME can be done anytime, anywhere, whenever you want to stop stress in its tracks and get quick intuitive access. As you practice, you'll learn to systematically weave heart intelligence into your daily life.

➤ A system of simple reminders to practice can help novices become fluent at FREEZE-FRAME. You can set digital alarms or post notes on a mirror, refrigerator, or computer screensaver, for example.

➤ Don't underestimate the power of neutral. The ability to find neutral, and stay put there until your heart shows you clearly what to do, is a sign of balance and maturity. The neutral state is a conduit for objectivity in the moment.

➤ FREEZE-FRAME offers you a scientifically researched, user-friendly method to add coherent heart power to whatever you do. The Heart-Math tools and techniques are designed to be facilitators of, not competitors with, personal development and spiritual growth methods.

# CHAPTER 5

# Energy Efficiency

The alarm clock goes off at 6:30 A.M., and before Steve even opens his eyes, unpleasant thoughts begin to take shape. "I hate getting up. I don't want to go to work. Today's going to be a real bear."

Steve drags himself into the shower as he continues to silently process a stream of concerns about leftover problems from yesterday and anxieties about today—his workload, the cold weather, and how burned out he feels.

"I'll be okay as soon as I get my cup of coffee," he assures himself as the warm shower begins to neutralize the shock of waking up. He gets dressed and goes downstairs, only to find that the automatic coffeemaker hasn't come on. There's no coffee brewed, and no time to start any now. "Damn, I can't believe this!" he says, slapping his hand on the counter as his emotions start to simmer.

On the way to work (with no coffee in hand), Steve turns on the radio and hears a talk-show host informing listeners about the rise in teenage drug use. He thinks about his own teenage son and how unusual he's been acting lately. Anxiety about the boy and his possible drug use begins to invade his commute. He pushes those thoughts aside and switches stations, only to hear that his favorite basketball team lost an important game the night before by just two points and has been eliminated from the playoffs. "What next?" he thinks.

When he arrives at work, the receptionist smiles and says, "Good morning, Steve. How are you?"

"Never better," he answers mechanically.

Near his office he spots a co-worker with whom he had a major conflict several days earlier. Irritation begins to build on cue. "That SOB," he mutters. "I'll get him back when he least expects it."

Once in his office, he listens to his voice-mail while starting up his computer to review a list of unanswered e-mails from the day before. Ten voice-mails, thirty e-mails. Steve is already feeling overloaded, and he's just getting started.

Surprisingly, though, the day goes pretty well. When he learns that a business deal he's been working on is moving forward, he feels a rush of excitement. A new client really impresses him, and he has an enjoyable conversation with her.

Just before lunch he has some sharp words with his secretary over an incomplete letter. While eating, he evaluates the incident and realizes that he hadn't given her enough information to do what he'd asked. Upon returning to the office, he apologizes. He feels good about having made that caring effort.

Later on a friendly co-worker stops by to thank him for a favor, and his spirit is further revived by this act of appreciation.

Steve leaves work feeling the way he often does—not great, but not lousy either. He has kind of a cardboard feeling—dull but not really bad.

Once home he greets his wife, who proceeds to tell him, at some length, that her sister has a health problem. The doctors don't know what it is yet, but she'll be going in for tests in a few days. As they start to discuss the possibilities, a variety of dire outcomes are projected.

As they sit down to dinner, Steve is feeling drained, but he tries to encourage himself with the prospect of his favorite TV show later on. Then his wife reminds him that their insurance agent is coming over in an hour to talk about upgrading their life insurance policy. As any chance for a break slips from his hands, Steve starts to complain. Although his level of tension has nothing to do with his wife, he exchanges terse words with her.

After the insurance agent finally leaves, it's time for bed. As his head hits the pillow, Steve is drained and exhausted. "At least tomorrow is Wednesday—hump day. A few more days and I'll have the weekend to relax."

Steve's experience is common for millions of people—successful people who have it made: a career, a family, a late-model car, reliable health. Despite their success, they're in survival mode emotionally. Their energy is depleted; they feel tired and overloaded. This largely unfulfilling quality of life results from not putting enough emphasis on managing thoughts and feelings.

As we look back at Steve's experience, how much of his internal dialogue came from mechanical, unmanaged head reactions and how much came from his heart? Was he using his mental and emotional energy efficiently or inefficiently? Which thoughts and feelings added to his quality of life and which produced stress?

Freeze-Frame, the technique that you learned in the previous chapter, is designed to address these issues, as are the "heart power tools" and Cut-Thru, which you'll learn about later. By using these tools and techniques to become more coherent, Steve would eliminate thoughts and feelings that drain his energy. He would also know how to consciously experience the kinds of thoughts and feelings that add energy to his system. Instead of establishing a depleting succession of emotions—a succession that gains momentum throughout the day—he would have the means to nip that pattern in the bud. Unfortunately, many of us live our lives completely unconscious of how we're spending our vital energy reserves. As a result, our health and happiness suffer.

Whether we're aware of it or not, an energy economy game is going on inside of us throughout life. Our inner experience over the course of each day includes thousands of thoughts, feelings, and impressions that directly impact our energy level. It's not easy to keep up with all of them, but if we're self-observant, we can catch ourselves when we're thinking and feeling in ways that deduct from our energy account and instead adopt attitudes and perspectives that give us a boost. Even in the midst of a major problem, when it's hard to appreciate much of anything, we can neutralize our reactions and come back to balance by easing into our hearts and using FREEZE-FRAME to shift our perspective.

This isn't to imply that we should see everything that happens to us each day as wonderful, covering over problems with a false veneer. But it's possible to face difficulties with equilibrium, to react to disappointments with wisdom and insight, and to see past our personal agendas when we interact with others. In other words, it's time for us to grow up. A mature approach to living means that we see problems for what they are without exaggerating their importance or sacrificing more important values to solve them.

## Quantum Nutrients

We're taught from childhood on to be very careful about what we put into our bodies. As early as elementary school, we learn that eating balanced meals is the key to proper nutrition. But the research we describe in this book shows that the thoughts and feelings we consume are equally, if not more, important. Our mental and emotional diets determine our overall energy levels, health, and well-being to a far greater extent than most people realize.

Physiologically speaking, when we experience stress our energy reserves are *redirected*. Processes that break down the body's energy stores for immediate use are activated at the *expense* of processes that maintain, repair, and regenerate our systems. The body's aim is to make energy available to help us confront our stressors. [1]

It comes down to a simple fact: when our energy reserves are continually channeled into the stress pathway, there isn't enough energy left to support regenerative processes that replenish the resources we've lost, repair damage to our bodies, and defend us against disease. The synthesis of new stores of protein, fats, and carbohydrates is halted; the repair and replacement of most kinds of cells is diminished; bone repair and wound healing is slowed; and levels of circulating immune cells and antibodies fall. [1] In the long run, as we saw in Chapter 3, stress depletes our system and can be severely damaging to our health.

Recent research suggests that high levels of emotional distress can even impair the crucial molecular repair processes that keep DNA damage in check. [2] And we know that in high levels the stress hormone cortisol kills our brain cells. [3]

On the other hand, each time we activate the power of our hearts and experience beneficial feelings such as sincere appreciation, care, and love, we're allowing the electrical energy of our hearts to work for us. Though our mood may visibly improve, the most powerful effects are generally invisible. When we consciously choose a core heart feeling over a negative feeling, we effectively intercept the physiological stress response that drains and damages our system and allow the body's natural regenerative capacities to work for us. Instead of being taxed and depleted, our mental and emotional systems are renewed. As a consequence, they're better able to ward off future "energy eaters"—stress, anxiety, and anger, for example—before they take hold.

As our entire system aligns with these beneficial emotions, we begin to experience a powerful new level of energy efficiency. What starts off as *psychological* nutrition becomes *physiological* at the most fundamental levels. There's greater cooperation and less friction between the two branches of the autonomic nervous system. This significantly lessens the wear and tear on the heart, the brain, and all the body's other organs, and heightens the efficiency with which the body performs the many functions that keep us alive and healthy. [4] Numerous studies have revealed that people who practice the HeartMath Solution tools and techniques to manage their mind and emotions and bring more core heart feelings into their everyday lives experience significantly less fatigue and greater physical energy and vitality. [5–9]

Heartfelt positive feelings create far more than a healthy psychological effect. They fortify our internal energy systems and nourish the body right down to the cellular level. For that reason, we like to think of these emotions as "quantum nutrients."

# Daily Reserves

The way we accumulate and spend our vital energy reserves is the primary factor that determines the quality of our lives. Most of us aren't used to associating our emotions with our energy level. We may be vaguely aware that when we're enthusiastic, our energy goes up. But how often do we associate the emotions we've experienced with how tired we feel at the end of the day?

If we have no energy left for the weekend after a stressful week, how often do we say, "Well, let's see. I let myself get angry twice on Tuesday and Wednesday; then I was consumed with worry about our deadline practically all day Thursday and Friday. With that kind of emotional mismanagement, no wonder I'm drained!"

Noticing our energy drains and gains requires a shift in awareness—and a little experimentation. But the energy boost that results will speak for itself.

Whether we like it or not, we're accountable for our energy expenditures. In physics, the law of conservation of energy states that energy can never be created or destroyed; it can only be changed from one form to another.

We wake up in the morning with a certain amount of vital energy to expend each day. It's up to us whether we expend it in efficient or nonefficient thoughts, feelings, and attitudes. As we've seen, allowing incoherence to reign in our bodies dissipates internal energy quickly, while coherence saves energy, keeping our systems in sync.

Nothing can happen without energy. For anything to move or change, energy is needed. When we understand how energy works in our mental, emotional, and physical systems, we can get our energy working *for* us rather than *against* us. When we drain energy through incoherence, we have to build back our energy reserves (just as we have to put more money in our checking account when we're overdrawn).

# Managing Our Energy Accounts

Many psychoanalysts consider money to be symbolic of the power and energy in our lives. In our consumer society, we tend to spend a lot of time thinking about money—how much money's coming in, how much is going out, how much we want in the future, and how much we've lost in the past.

Sociologists say that to be successful adults in the world today—to run our own lives—we have to master skills that used to apply only to bankers, administrators, and time-management specialists. While some people don't balance their checkbooks or pay off at least the minimum on their credit cards, most of us have grown accustomed to monitoring our cash flow and expenditures to keep our accounts balanced. Why not apply these same skills to our energy management?

Think about it this way. What if we had an inner computer—a heart computer—that could calculate every thought, feeling, and emotion? Suppose it logged each one, determining whether it added or took away energy and assessing how much it increased or depleted our vitality, and then provided a readout that represented our available energy reserves.

In a sense, this inner computer exists. Every thought and feeling, no matter how big or small, *does* impact our inner energy reserves. And at any given moment, our physiological state reflects the status of our account.

We can learn to monitor and manage our energy bank account, keeping track of our deposits and withdrawals to ensure a growing "net worth." When we start paying attention to our energy account, it's the glaring expenditures that we notice first. Was it really worth it to get so worked up over petty frustrations at the office that we felt tired and agitated during our precious moments at home? After all, quality time isn't *quality* if we're struggling to recover from stress.

It's certainly important to eliminate extravagant expenditures on stress that overdraw our energy account—expenditures such as fuming all the way home at that driver who insisted on driving ten miles under the speed limit and wouldn't pull off the road to let us pass. But as we practice listening to our hearts, we'll start to notice even the little things that drain us.

Those small emotional indulgences—worry, guilt, and judgments of ourselves or others, for example—cost a lot more than we realize. When it comes to money, we're all familiar with the impact of those small, apparently harmless daily expenditures. Though we don't generally include such expenditures in the budget, we know that spending a couple dollars a day on a cappuccino or a magazine to flip through at lunch adds up fast. And if we're a hundred dollars short for car repairs at the end of the month, we know where to look: at the accumulation of insidious little things we hardly think about.

Recently, Deborah Rozman, one of our associates, was giving a FREEZE-FRAME workshop to the entire staff of a major TV network talk show, including the producers, bookers, camera people, and writers. The hosts were going to interview her on air the next day and wanted to first experience the FREEZE-FRAME technique for themselves.

During the training, each person filled out an energy asset/deficit balance sheet—we'll come to those in a minute—to determine efficient and nonefficient energy expenditures over the previous three days. Afterwards they discussed the results.

Since these participants knew that TV was a high-stress profession, deadline following deadline, it didn't surprise them that their energy deficits outweighed their assets. They could *feel* it. But what they didn't realize was that most of their energy deficits were centered not around work deadlines but around relationships, communication problems, money worries, and judgments.

One of the hosts said, "You know, my life feels like that movie *Groundhog Day*. Each morning I get up and I see the same day ahead of me. Each night I go to bed thinking something's got to change.

"I don't feel the textures of life you're talking about. In fact, I feel numb most of the time. How do you get off this hamster-wheel existence? Quit work and move to the country?"

In the lively discussion that followed, most of the staff said they felt exactly the same way. Until then, they'd attributed the feeling to the nature of their jobs and to life in New York City. But even librarians in small-town America complain that stress is draining them until they're numb.

We can't blame the stimulation of workplace or city; it's the *internal environment* of irritation, frustration, anger, blame, and judgment that creates our stress and causes the heart to shut down. Our core heart feelings are cut off when judgments or blame dominate, and then we can no longer feel the nurturing textures of life. When we're out of touch with appreciation, care, and love, life becomes dry and stressful and the mind functions mechanically, without intuition or clarity.

So if quitting our jobs and moving to the country isn't the answer, what is? What can we do to put quality back into our lives? The first step is to get a readout from our heart computer. If we could see how much energy we waste through a single negative emotional state—say, judgment—in just one week, we'd be surprised.

Then, once we know our state of mind and heart, we can move forward. All it takes is noticing those judgments (or worries or feelings of guilt) as they happen and consciously replacing them with appreciation, compassion, and tolerance in the moment. That simple act of "conversion" stops the energy drain and restores regenerative power. Having taken that step, we can then ease our way gradually back to the heart.

Most of the stress overload we feel is nothing more than the taxes we're paying on inefficient mental and emotional energy management. We can try to blame the events and people in our lives for the way we feel. Yet we're the ones who spent too long at the computer without a break or pushed through the day on adrenaline and willpower alone, instead of stopping to build up our reserves. If we'd take a minute every so often to do a FREEZE-FRAME and engage the power of the heart, we could make energy adjustments moment by moment that would reduce the effects of overload.

## Becoming Our Own Accountants

As we've seen, some of our thoughts and emotional responses are assets that contribute energy to our system, while others are deficits that deplete and drain us. Some of these assets and deficits are subtle; some are obvious. Some are relatively neutral; others are extreme. But *all* of our inner dialogues, thought processes, and feeling states fall generally into either the asset or the deficit category.

Clearly, if we're accumulating more assets than deficits, our energy account is growing in value. A healthy reserve of assets results in vitality, adaptability, resiliency, creativity, and a steady improvement in a healthy quality of life—psychologically and physically.

If, on the other hand, our deficits accrue faster than our assets, our energy account is diminishing in value. We become emotionally spent and wear out more quickly. Our creativity, productivity, and available intelligence diminish, as does our ability to roll with the punches while keeping a hopeful and positive perspective. If we're accumulating more deficits than assets, our quality of life decreases significantly.

Let's look at a typical energy deficit. When we have an argument with a good friend, the experience takes a lot out of us. After the harsh words have been said and the dust has settled, we feel tired more than anything. Our energy has been noticeably depleted. It can take days to recover from an argument—especially if we continue to replay the incident over and over in our heads. And if we make a practice of that sort of replay analysis, our long-term health will suffer.

Though we may notice that we feel especially tired after an argument, we rarely stop and reflect on what took place in our bodies during that time. Recent research gives us an inside look at what our inner systems are doing while we're busy criticizing, complaining, or blaming.

Psychologist Janice Kiecolt-Glaser and immunologist Ronald Glaser of Ohio State University looked at the effects of abrasive marital interactions on heart rate, blood pressure, hormonal, and immune system health. When married couples discussed sensitive issues in the laboratory, those who were most hostile in their interchanges experienced not only an elevated heart rate and a significant rise in blood pressure, but also a marked increase in stress hormones and a drop-off in immunity that was still evident when the couple left the research center the next day. Interactions characterized by hostility, criticism, sarcasm, and blame—indicating a refusal to take responsibility and demeaning the other partner—proved to be the most damaging.

These effects occurred despite the fact that the subjects said they were highly satisfied in their marriages, led healthy lifestyles, and were in optimal physical health. Moreover, whether the couples were newlyweds or had been married for over forty years didn't matter; similar physiological responses were observed. [10–12]

It's not hard to see how these results tie in with the data from long-term studies showing that people who are typically angry, hostile, and aggressive tend to have increased rates of heart disease and premature death later in life. [13, 14]

Were we to stop and consider the barrage of damaging physiological responses to which we expose ourselves each time we argue, we might think twice about whether it was worth it.

On the other hand, when we have a meaningful conversation with another person and feel a true sense of agreement—a strong connection and rapport of the heart—we're invigorated. Time seems to fly by: it's 3:00 A.M., but we still feel energized! And the energy endures long after the good-byes have been said. Each time we think about that conversation over the next few days, we feel a sense of buoyancy and regeneration. During positive interactions such as that, we experience many of the positive emotions that stimulate our immune system to fend off invaders more readily [15] and allow our various bodily systems to communicate more easily. [4] Clearly, conversations that energize us are assets.

For the next few days, observe your communications with others to see where they're energizing and where they're draining. Appreciate those that are energizing as they're happening; that additional positive response actually adds more energy to your bank account. In difficult, draining communications, ease into the heart and find something to appreciate about the person you're with, or find a feeling of compassion or kindness. Looking for the good won't turn you into a doormat. It will clear your mind and give you the coherence you need to know what to say next. That's energy efficiency at work.

The HeartMath Solution tools and techniques—FREEZE-FRAME and others that we'll learn about throughout this book—are designed to generate emotional and mental coherence deliberately, on demand, so that we can spend more time at this optimal, regenerative level of energy efficiency.

Learning to maintain a diet high in quality thoughts and feelings contributes significantly to our energy and to the elimination of stress. Every time a negative mind activity of any kind is stopped and heart intelligence is activated, energy accumulates. With repetition of this process over time, we're rejuvenated mentally, emotionally, and physically.

We tell children to "just say no" to strangers, drugs, certain foods, and other threats to their health or safety. But as adults we often have a hard time saying no to some of the most damaging influences we're confronted with—our negative thoughts, attitudes, and emotions. We experience inner turmoil or vent our feelings at others because we don't want to repress them.

But research has shown that energy drain takes place in the presence of these negative mental and emotional states either way, whether we vent them or repress them; if we *have* them, we can't win. So we have to go one step further: if we don't *engage* the frustration, anger, judgment, or blame, we don't have anything to vent or repress. But learning how not to engage takes new intelligence, maturity, and power.

Earlier in this chapter we mentioned the energy asset/deficit balance sheet. This is an excellent self-management strategy for monitoring how much vital energy you're spending and saving. Keeping a written record of your energy assets and deficits is well worth the time it takes. Keeping an inventory even for a few days will give you an extremely clear picture of where you're adding to (or withdrawing from) your energy account, and how you're doing it. You'll be able to see which mental/emotional patterns are beneficial to your well-being and which are not.

## Asset/Deficit Balance Sheet

Try tracking your energy deposits and withdrawals over a twenty-four period—either today or yesterday, so that it's fresh in your mind—on the asset/deficit balance sheet found on page 97. First think back over the day

# Asset/Deficit Balance Sheet

*Under Assets*, list the positive events, conversations, and interactions of a specific time. List as many assets as you can think of, feeling appreciation for each asset as you go. Also list *ongoing* assets in your life—overall quality of friends, family, living and/or working environment, etc. (Notice how conscious you were of these assets during the period.)

*Under Deficits*, list issues, conflicts, and events that were negative or draining during that same period.

| Points | Assets | | Deficits | Points |
|---|---|---|---|---|
| _____ | _____ | | _____ | _____ |
| _____ | _____ | **Issues to Consider** | _____ | _____ |
| _____ | _____ | | _____ | _____ |
| _____ | _____ | Alignment with Core Values | _____ | _____ |
| _____ | _____ | | _____ | _____ |
| _____ | _____ | Effect on Family/Work | _____ | _____ |
| _____ | _____ | | _____ | _____ |
| _____ | _____ | Stressful/ Nonstressful | _____ | _____ |
| _____ | _____ | | _____ | _____ |
| _____ | _____ | People Involved | _____ | _____ |
| _____ | _____ | | _____ | _____ |
| _____ | _____ | Feelings | _____ | _____ |
| _____ | _____ | | _____ | _____ |

_____ **Assets Total**    _____**Total Score**    **Deficits Total** _____

After listing assets and deficits, step back and, from the heart, compare lists. Evaluate which deficits could still be transformed into assets. Notice which deficits could have been neutralized or turned into assets *at the time* had you stopped long enough to gain a wider perspective.

**Conclusions:** _____

_____

_____

_____

_____

you're auditing. As objectively as possible—trying not to overidentify with right or wrong, good or bad—think about the flow of the day. Then follow these instructions:

1. Under "Assets," write down the events that were energizing and harmonious, that felt good to your system. These may include such things as enjoyable interactions with others, acts of kindness, times when you could have become upset but didn't, or creative time by yourself.

2. Under "Deficits," write down the events that felt incoherent, disharmonious, or draining. These may include miscommunications, overreactions, frustrations, worries, time pressures, or inefficient uses of your energy—anything that didn't feel good to you.

3. When you're through listing these events, put +1 by each asset and –1 by each deficit. Then add up your assets, add up your deficits, and subtract the deficits from the assets to determine your overall score. If you're in the red, it's time to take action.

What did you learn from doing this exercise? Did you see more clearly how your attitudes and perspectives contributed to how you felt on the day that was audited? Did you see repetitive patterns—things that you do regularly that added to or subtracted from your score? Were there some deficits that you wanted to assign a lower score—a –5 or –50 instead of just –1—because of how much they upset or drained you? Were there some assets that you wanted to score higher because of the extra energy or fun they gave you? Perhaps you had events on your sheet that were *both* assets and deficits. This isn't uncommon. Some events combine positive and negative feeling states—for example, an outing to the mall with your son that started out great but ended in argument.

Did you see events in your deficit column that could have become assets with just a little more heart effort to manage your reaction and do something differently? Did you see deficits that could easily have been eliminated or even transformed into assets by using FREEZE-FRAME?

As you recalled your day, did you weigh the deficit events more heavily than the assets, thinking that your day was worse than it actually was? Don't worry. Most people do. Ignoring the assets and dwelling on the deficits is one of the head's favorite tricks.

Are there assets you could have appreciated more at the time (or would like to appreciate more in general)? We often take our assets for granted. As we noted earlier, stopping to appreciate an asset accumulates even more energy, giving us a buffer that helps us take in stride the lumps and bumps of daily stressors.

Regardless of the total score you assigned yourself, the act of caring enough about your own personal development to take an inventory of your energy expenditures is a big asset. Most people won't slow down enough to be conscious about how they're spending their energy. You did—and in our opinion that's worth at least five asset points in itself!

Keeping an asset/deficit balance sheet is a first step toward freedom. Writing down and numerically scoring your energy management will refine your awareness and help you become more energy-efficient. As you become more sensitive to your thoughts and feelings, you'll naturally start to use your heart to oversee your energy consumption and build up your power.

## Powering Up Your Life

The bottom line is this: when your energy accumulators stay full, you have more power to accomplish your personal goals, deflect stress, eliminate self-defeating behaviors, and increase awareness. When your accumulators are depleted, life is harder, awareness is numbed, change is hard to make, and you don't feel satisfied (much less happy and fulfilled). Which way would *you* rather live?

The HeartMath Solution formula for building the power you need to make the changes you want is simple: *Stop energy drains and infuse your system with free energy as you go.* In colloquial terms we might say, Fill your bucket, but first plug the holes. When your energy accumulators are full, events and situations that would previously have bothered or stressed you are more easily seen as opportunities. If you apply heart first, your head can get in sync with your heart intelligence.

By using your heart as your compass, you can see more clearly which direction to go to stop self-defeating behavior. If you take just one thing that really bothers or drains you and apply heart intelligence to it, you'll see a noticeable difference in your life.

Review your asset/deficit balance sheet and study asset patterns that you'd like to enhance and deficit patterns that you'd like to change. Add to your balance sheet other assets and deficits that commonly occur but didn't come up on the day you audited. You might, for example, want to add to your asset list a dear friend whom you appreciate deeply and write to often, a favorite hobby that brings you peace, or special times with your child that bring you joy. On your deficit list, add anything that repeatedly drains your account—perhaps an obsession, a repetitive reaction to another person, a tendency to worry, or something you do without thinking about the consequences (such as getting angry while driving the car). Pick one deficit at a time to apply heart power to, practice the FREEZE-FRAME technique on, and get an intuitive perspective for. Then follow your heart's directives. See how much you can accomplish. You might be surprised.

There's a bonus to be had in addressing key issues that are obvious energy deficits. They're often nexus points that relate to other problems. A lot of patterns conjoin at one spot, in one underlying basic pattern. So changing one often opens the door for a release of free energy that floods you with the power to more easily shift other attitudes and behaviors.

Making internal and external changes takes power. Trying to figure things out with your head alone results in a lot of incoherent mental pushing and pulling—an energy expenditure that just isn't necessary when you come from the heart. Because the head is linear, the steps it takes to work things out are necessarily incremental. If you run out of energy along the way, you may forsake the quest before you reach the goal.

Creating a joint venture between head and heart puts a power pack behind your goals. Getting your head in sync with your heart and harnessing the power of coherence gives you the energy efficiency you need to achieve changes that haven't been possible before. The head can notice what things need to change, but the heart provides the power and direction to actually bring about the changes.

Recognizing your energy assets and deficits, paying close attention to your inner dialogue, and using the heart's guidance to increase your asset-to-deficit ratio is one of the fastest ways we know of to accumulate the energy needed to make quantum leaps in becoming the person you want to be.

## KEY POINTS TO REMEMBER

➤ Our mental and emotional diets determine our overall energy levels, health, and well-being to a far greater extent than most people realize. Every thought and feeling, no matter how big or small, impacts our inner energy reserves.

➢ Look at life as an energy economy game. Each day, ask yourself, "Are my energy expenditures (actions, reactions, thoughts, and feelings) productive or nonproductive? During the course of my day, have I accumulated more stress or more peace?"

➢ Keeping an asset/deficit balance sheet even for a few days will give you an extremely clear picture of where you're adding to your energy account, where you're overdrawing it, and how you're accomplishing both.

➢ When we consciously evoke core heart feelings, we nourish our bodies at every level. Like quantum nutrients, core heart feelings keep our cells regenerating.

➢ Learning to "just say no" to emotional reactions isn't repression. Saying no means not *engaging* the frustration, anger, judgment, or blame. Without engagement, you won't have anything to repress.

➢ The goal of HeartMath is to help you learn to generate emotional and mental coherence deliberately—on demand—so that ultimately you spend more of your day at this optimal, regenerative level of energy efficiency.

➢ In communications that are difficult or draining, ease into the heart and find something to appreciate about the person you're dealing with, or find a feeling of compassion or kindness. This will clear your mind and give you the coherence you need to know what to say next. That's energy efficiency at work.

➢ By using your heart as your compass, you can see more clearly which direction to go to stop self-defeating behavior. If you take just one mental or emotional habit that really bothers or drains you and apply heart intelligence to it, you'll see a noticeable difference in your life.

# CHAPTER 6

# At the Heart's Core:
# The Power Tools of the Heart

Papa John lived at the edge of town amid the corn and tobacco fields in a small red-brick house. Driving the beat-up old truck he used to make his living, he would show up at the houses and businesses in our small town once or twice a week to collect the trash and haul it to the dump. We always liked to see him coming, a big smile on his face and his eyes gleaming with kindness. Every interaction, no matter how brief, left us feeling as if we'd been touched with goodness and honor.

Papa John was well known in our North Carolina town of six hundred people. Rich or poor, young or old, black or white, people loved and respected him. What was it about this lovable black man that gave him such a warm and generous personality? What was it that transcended social status and race to gently win our hearts?

Papa John's secret was appreciation. You could tell by looking at him, by watching his interactions with people and things, that he walked through life in a state of deep, sincere appreciation. He appreciated every little thing in life—the way the sun was shining and the birds were singing, the way his wife made his lunch just as he liked it, the way his customers greeted him by name. Even on the days when his seventy-five-year-old body didn't want to respond to the call of his youthful spirit, he never let it get him down. Rain or shine, hot or cold, late or early, he was always smiling, eager to reach out to shake your hand and caringly ask how you were doing that day.

When we told him that we were moving to California, it was clear that his words of kindness all those years had been genuine. But despite (and through) his sadness, he let us know that if he couldn't appreciate seeing us every week, he'd still appreciate having known us at all. He'd filled his heart up with appreciation for so long that he could return to that emotion from sadness with incredible grace and ease.

His simple, appreciative presence was so endearing that, after we settled in California, we flew Papa John out for a visit. We'd been thinking about him a lot—missing him—and we wanted our colleagues at the Institute to meet him.

Among our staff of business professionals and scientists, Papa John worked the same magic he had in North Carolina. Within a day, everybody wanted to be around him.

As he was getting into the car that would take him to the airport, surrounded by a group of us, he smiled at each individual in turn—that smile that lit up his whole face. "There are a lot of problems in the world," he said, "but now, when anybody asks, I can say I know where there's a piece of heaven. It's right here with all of you."

Looked at in some ways, Papa John's life had been harder than most. He had a job that few people would want. The house he lived in wasn't much to speak of. And he never had money to burn. But the level of appreciation he radiated into the world was more valuable by far than success or riches. He'd cultivated one of the heart's most precious qualities: wherever he went, he connected powerfully to the world with love. And people responded.

Core heart feelings—including appreciation, care, compassion, nonjudgment, and forgiveness—are very potent. They're all aspects of love. In this chapter we'll discuss three of these qualities—those we call "heart power tools": appreciation, nonjudgment, and forgiveness. In a later chapter we'll present a fourth heart power tool: care. These qualities come from the depth of our being—from the core of the heart. Activating core heart feelings increases energy assets and reduces or eliminates energy deficits. Properly directed, these feelings can change our lives—and perhaps the world.

But we don't have time for such nonsense, right? "These are sweet concepts," some might say, "but life is too hard to accommodate them. People with a soft touch teach us about loving our neighbors and forgiving in Sunday school, but everybody knows life doesn't really work that way." Heart-based qualities sound appealing, to be sure, but they don't seem *real* enough to be useful when we're dealing with tough issues such as job security, relationships, finances, or health.

Ironically, we react this way to heart-based qualities not because they don't apply to our problems in the real world but because we lack a practical *way* to apply them. Now that even science has shown us how incredibly good these core heart feelings are for our bodies and minds—as we've seen in preceding chapters—it's time to transfer them from the sky to the street, from airy-fairy concepts to down-to-earth reality.

As I (Doc) have often said, "We're about the business of the heart. From the moment we started looking into the power of the heart, we've been interested not in sentiment but in what *works*.

"That's why I don't hesitate to call such tender feelings as care or appreciation 'power tools.' It seems kind of jarring to some, but I want to emphasize the point: these aren't just nice sensations meant to put us in a better mood. They have *muscle*. Once you see the results, you'll understand why the name 'power tools' is appropriate."

## Sincerity

Taken by itself, a random feeling of appreciation or care doesn't mean much. Sure, it's nice. A good moment. Better, in that instant, than feeling stress. But "powerful"? No.

Remember, the main difference between the light coming from a laser beam and that coming from a sixty-watt bulb is coherence. In order to turn emotions that we barely notice into high-powered tools, we've got to learn to apply them with *focused* intention and consistency. Only then will we see their energy efficiency and tangible results.

A scientist in a lab who fires up his laser beam can approach his job in any mood at all. Whether he does it enthusiastically, halfheartedly, or with a downright bad attitude, when he flips the power switch the laser beam turns on.

For some reason, nature didn't design core heart feelings like that. To power them up, sincerity is essential. Sincerity motivates our heart and aligns our true intentions. Sincerity is the generator that brings core heart feelings into coherence and gives them power.

To derive coherence from these power tools, we must be motivated by a sincere desire. Our heart knows the difference. We all had times as kids when we were forced, against our better judgment, to apologize to someone for something we'd done. With our parents looking grimly over our shoulder, we mouthed the words, but we didn't mean them. Maybe our parents fell for it. Maybe the recipient of the apology did too. But there wasn't a single cell in our own bodies that believed it. We *knew* we weren't sincere. And now, as we face the opportunity to develop power tools of the heart, there's no one looking over our shoulder but our heart—and again our heart will know.

A practical first step, if you have any doubts about the potential of these power tools, is to ask your heart whether loving, appreciating, and forgiving could really do anything for you. If you get the feeling that they might, you'll find it easier to give these tools a try with sincerity.

The more sincerity you can muster when applying the heart power tools, the more power they'll have. You'll soon find that these familiar feelings take on new life. The amount of benefit you receive will be in direct proportion to the amount of sincerity you apply.

## Heart Power Tools

### Power Tool 1: Appreciation

People like Papa John who are naturally appreciative have a glow about them. It's not that their life has fewer challenges, but nothing seems to get them down; and they have a greater ability to bounce back when things don't go their way. That's because appreciation is highly magnetic and energizing.

Generally, appreciation means some blend of thankfulness, admiration, approval, and gratitude. In the financial world, something that "appreciates" grows in value. With the power tool of appreciation, you get the benefit of both perspectives: as you learn to be consistently thankful and approving, your life will grow in value.

As you'll remember from Chapter 2, participants in a research study created an efficient, healthy state of entrainment—depicted in the coherent heart rhythms shown on Figure 2.5—by deliberately generating a feeling of appreciation. In that state of entrainment, the two main branches of the autonomic nervous system are synchronized, enjoying just enough stimulation and just enough relaxation. Appreciation is a powerful force. It eats the stress response for breakfast.

You can be confident that as you focus on sincere feelings of appreciation, your nervous system will naturally come into balance. Biologically, all of the systems in your body, including your brain, will work in greater harmony. The electromagnetic field radiating from your body will resonate with the ordered, coherent pattern emitted by your heart. And every cell in your system will benefit.

With your body in an improved state of balance, you'll start to feel better emotionally—and it's no wonder. Just as appreciation causes the jagged heart rhythms on the graph to relax into an even flow, so your thoughts and feelings begin to interact more smoothly.

Appreciation has a way of smoothing out life's lumps and bumps. It puts things into perspective, reducing the heaviness and density of stressful thoughts and feelings. In a moment of sincere appreciation, your day no longer feels like the burden it used to be. You're free to see and acknowledge the good things in life for a change.

Opening your heart is like putting a wide-angle lens on the camera of your perception. Suddenly, more of the world comes into view. You have more room for new possibilities in the picture.

And keep in mind that like attracts like. An electromagnetic field is just that: magnetic. The emotional resonance you send out from your coherent heart rhythms is like a magnet, attracting people, situations, and opportunities. When you're in a state of appreciation, your energy is more buoyant and spirited. You feel better mentally, emotionally, and physically.

### What If I Don't Feel Like It?

The great thing about appreciation is that it's generally a much easier feeling to generate than love or care. Let's say you're having the day from hell. Every single thing you've touched has gone wrong. People you hadn't expected to hear from have called to tell you things you didn't want to know. Every piece of machinery you've gotten within ten feet of—including the wretched phone—has malfunctioned. You're on the verge of pulling out your hair when you remember to use the power tool of appreciation.

When you're in the grip of that sort of frustration, love seems out of the question. Even care is a big stretch. But appreciation is easy—even if it starts out tinged with sarcasm: "I appreciate the fact that I haven't fallen flat on my face . . . yet." After a couple of stabs at it, you're going to stumble across something that sincerely touches you. Maybe it's your friends, your partner, your loved ones. And all it takes is one strong dose of appreciation to turn your perceptions around 180 degrees.

Last year a friend of ours, Brent, went through a terrible divorce. The fighting and bickering raged on for months. When we stopped by to see him one day, he'd just hung up after a volatile, contentious phone call from his estranged wife. He was in the depths of despair. We tried to talk to him, but nothing we said had an impact.

While we were talking with Brent, his five-year-old son came over and leaned against him. He looked at his father tenderly and said, "Daddy, I really love you." Then he walked out of the room. Brent's smile was priceless. Once his son had reminded him of how much love and appreciation they felt for each other, he realized that nothing else really mattered. The tension and stress he'd felt from that phone call evaporated before our eyes.

### Losing Power by Adapting

If only we could depend on life to bring us those wonderful bursts of appreciation, we wouldn't have to develop the skill of finding it on our own. We could just kick back and wait for it to fall into our laps. No matter how miserable we felt, we could tell ourselves, "Any moment now, my life is going to surprise me with something so sweet that I won't be able to resist appreciating it!" Well, maybe.

But chances are you're going to have to make the effort to notice something good yourself. And then you'll have to let go of the temptation to cling to misery. And *then*, once you feel appreciation, you'll have to learn to hang onto it, because the easiest thing in the world is to adapt to our habitual ways of thinking and feeling.

Suppose you buy one of the hottest new cars on the market—a sleek, black BMW loaded with so many technological marvels that it not only provides an interactive map of where you are, it practically picks your destination. This car is *cool*. Everybody wants it, but it's yours.

For a month or so, you get excited every time you see it sitting in the driveway. Without even intending to, you wash it twice a week. But after a few months—before that new car smell has even worn off—it's not as exciting anymore. It's *familiar*. You still love it, but the thrill is gone. Adaptation has set in.

Need we even mention relationships? Remember those early days of a special relationship when the other person was all that you could think of? Nothing else remotely compared to being with your girl (or guy). From the moment you parted, you couldn't wait to see her again. The connection was 100 percent engaging. But it waned. The infatuation didn't last, though the love, affection, and satisfaction may still remain decades later.

In the case of relationships, the adaptation that takes us past those giddy early stages of infatuation can open the door to a deeper connection. Even if we acknowledge, in those early stages, that all that glitters isn't gold, we're so enamored of the glitter that it's hard to distinguish the substance. As enjoyable as new relationships are, we can't love the other person for who he or she really is while we're blinded by infatuation. But once we grow into a deeper, more mature stage of our relationship, we can begin to appreciate that person in a new, rewarding way. It's an ever-changing process.

Adaptation isn't bad per se. But adaptation that causes us to drift instead of staying focused on our development or nod off instead of being awake diminishes our power for growth.

Say you have a major insight about something you want to change in your life. You get inspired and excited about what you're going to do. You start to implement your insight and make good headway for a week or two. You appreciate every accomplishment along the way. "I'm so glad that I decided to do this," you tell yourself.

After a while, though, you start to adapt; and as you do so, you begin to lose appreciation. You take your accomplishments and new insight for granted and tend not to be as consistent in your efforts. Your desire to sustain and complete the change you set out to make starts to fade. What's happening? You're allowing adaptation to eat away at your appreciation, cutting you off from the heart power needed to complete your efforts.

People who start out to accomplish changes more often than not don't carry them through to completion. This is especially true when what they're trying to change involves attitudes, ways of thinking, and emotional behavior. We've probably all had the experience of feeling our initial passion for a change wane—and then losing the impetus for change altogether. The initial heart directive that inspired us gets lost in day-to-day mind processing. Sometimes we have to go back and reactivate our commitment to earlier realizations until we have a progressive momentum going—and then we can supplement our initial appreciation with appreciation of the progress we've made!

By rekindling appreciation, we can bring things right back to the initial excitement we once had about our insight for change. Appreciation is a fire that resists dousing; it fights against adaptation until we've completed what we set out to do. Some things are worth rolling up our sleeves and revisiting because of the high payoff.

Maintaining an appreciative state takes consistent, conscious contact with our heart power—which bring us back to appreciating all that we already have, especially the little things.

### Deepening Appreciation

All of us have experienced events that were unpleasant at the time but that we later came to appreciate. On the simplest level, the drudgery of practice comes to mind. Children notoriously complain about practicing scales when they're taking music lessons. They don't want to *practice*; they just want to *play*. Nothing is more tedious than scales, but the work we put into them pays off in the end. On the night of a performance, an accomplished musician appreciates all those earlier hours of tedium.

One of the signs of maturity is our ability as adults to delay gratification, to do something we don't want to do right now in order to get something later that we *do* want. As we mature, we develop an increasing capacity to patiently endure temporary discomforts in order to reach the goals we prize the most. We also come to realize that not everything can be taken at face value.

While we sometimes *deliberately* delay gratification, at other times gratification comes unannounced—a pleasant surprise. Many events that cause us grief and pain, for example, ultimately bring unexpected rewards. Loss can open the door to whole new horizons. Disappointment can illuminate the road to success. With 20/20 hindsight—and a little distance from the pain—we often come to appreciate what we thought was a disaster.

Although we've all experienced this kind of "cloud with a silver lining," it's hard to approach painful events with appreciation in the moment. If your business folds or someone you care about rejects you, appreciation isn't the first thing that comes to mind. Wallowing in grief or pain seems natural in such cases—and natural it is.

Crying and kicking your feet is natural for an infant. But we grow out of that. Thinking that it's the end of the world if you're not popular at school is natural for a fourteen-year-old. But we grow out of that. Going into a funk when your life takes an unexpected turn for the worse is natural for an adult. But we can grow out of that too. Maturation is a natural process as well, and it's better in every way than the alternative.

The real challenge in using appreciation as a power tool is taking it to a deeper level. That means shifting to appreciation closer to the moment you learn about an apparent disaster. Now some of you are probably thinking, "If I can do that, I'm just a step away from walking on water!" But it's not as hard as it sounds.

Remember, appreciation is one of the easiest things to feel. All you have to do is access that emotion—no matter how bleak things seem at the start. Your heart will do the rest. If you can inject a hint of appreciation into your system in a moment of crisis, you've done your part. Just feel grateful for something, *anything*, in that moment. Your heart intelligence will respond accordingly. Then watch and learn.

For me (Doc), the trial by fire came many years ago when I joined the National Guard. From the moment I arrived at boot camp in Monterey, California, I hated it. Roll call at 5:00 A.M., bad food, and ten-mile hikes in the broiling sun with full packs. All day long, the drill sergeants treated us like dirt. I'd never expected to find myself scrubbing the floor of the latrine for hours on end with the only toothbrush I had! Try as I might, I could find nothing to appreciate about boot camp in the early days.

But gradually I began to notice little things I could appreciate, and once a little appreciation was found, it was easier to be glad for other things. As an example, when we were out doing maneuvers in miserable heat one day, the sergeant gave us a couple minutes of rest. Hot and sweaty, I stretched out on the ground to ease my aching muscles. My head landed on a little bed of ice plant that I hadn't noticed. On a day like that, it felt like a soft pillow, and I was grateful. My appreciation softened my heart. Instead of focusing through the lens of my own little aches, pains, and discomforts, I began to see the world through a lens of appreciation. Looking at the soldiers all around me, I realized how many new friends I was making as we went through this rite of manhood together.

I even came to have a certain appreciation for those tough-as-nails sergeants who were teaching us the skills we needed to survive. One time in particular comes to mind. In a classroom setting, someone was explaining how to use a compass to navigate in the woods. A few of us toward the back were messing around, not paying attention (as usual). The master sergeant caught on and had us do pushups until we were exhausted. As we grunted our way through the punishment, he yelled at us and called us every profane name imaginable. "What a jerk!" we thought.

A few days later, while on maneuvers, some of us got so lost that it took us miles and hours of extra walking through heavy, thorn-laden brush to finally make it back to camp—tired, starving, and bleeding. I could appreciate those sergeants pushing us to our limit in a whole new way after that.

The more things I learned to appreciate at boot camp, the more things I found to appreciate. By the end, I didn't want to leave. I'd found a way to make peace with boot camp that made even its most strenuous aspects fun. Looking back on it now, I can honestly say that it was one of the most fun and important experiences of my life. I didn't get to that place by repressing my true feelings or simply minimizing the bad and focusing on the good. I got there by starting with the few things I could sincerely appreciate; and from there my capacity to appreciate things I'd hated grew.

You can have that same experience in whatever challenging circumstances you find yourself, even if you've never tried it before. Appreciation is amazingly potent. It can take the edges off even the toughest situations.

### Appreciation in Action

Let's start with the exercise on page 112. Think of a situation in your life right now that's challenging. Calm the mind as much as you can by focusing in the area around the heart. Do a FREEZE-FRAME if you'd like. Ask your heart to show you three things about this situation to appreciate. Write them down.

Even if you didn't come up with a lot to appreciate, you've put a process into motion that will save you time and energy. By doing this exercise, you've time-shifted in a sense—brought the appreciation that you might later have come to naturally into the moment as best you could. This act of appreciating, even when it isn't an obvious time for appreciation, will help you resolve your challenging situation much more quickly and will increase your energy assets. Use appreciation not just when it's convenient but as a tool to help you see a way out of undesirable situations.

You can never get to peace and inner security without first acknowledging all of the good things in your life. If you're forever wanting and longing for more without first appreciating things the way they are, you'll stay in discord.

When your mind is unmanaged, it tends to focus on what's not right. And when you're caught up in your problems, focusing on what's not right, you tend to lose sight of areas in your life that are good. The result is that you end up feeling sorry for yourself. This kind of victimized thinking blocks off heart intelligence and creates perceptions that are narrow and confused. The way out is to activate appreciation and see the wider picture. If you stop and view your life from the heart, you'll find many things to appreciate. By doing this, you'll see things from a more balanced perspective. In other words, weighing a problem against the many things you can find to appreciate (if you look with the heart) lessens the significance of the problem. This is one of the magical ways in which appreciation works.

Now let's take a moment to fill in the appreciation list on page 113. Do a short FREEZE-FRAME and then list as many things as you can that you appreciate about your life. When you're finished, read your list and observe how this simple exercise makes you feel.

Creating an appreciation list gives you a new reference point for appreciation. Most of us don't take the time to inventory our blessings, but it's good practice.

# Appreciation Exercise

Challenging situation

Three things about this situation to appreciate

① 

② 

③

# Appreciation List

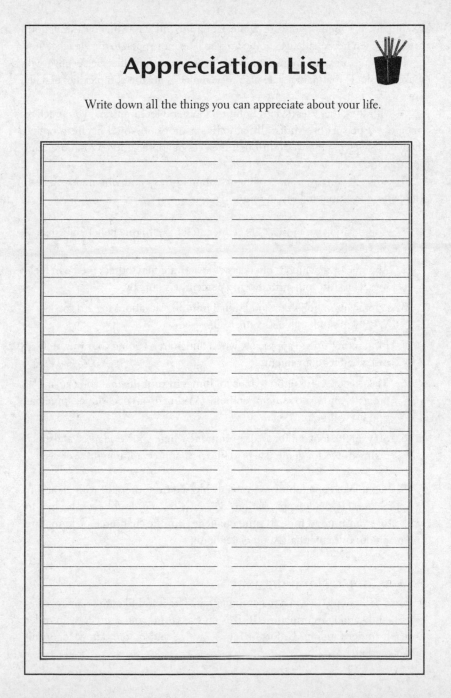

Write down all the things you can appreciate about your life.

Eventually, the memory of your appreciation list will stay with you throughout the day. When new challenges come up, you'll be more open to the idea that they could end up on your appreciation list before long. And that perspective will make it easier to maintain a state of appreciation despite the complexities of daily life.

As with the other HeartMath Solution tools and techniques, if you practice sincerely, a perspective shift will naturally occur. Soon you'll begin to notice that you're viewing the world through the eyes of appreciation a lot more than you used to.

Try to keep your awareness of appreciation as fresh and vibrant as you can. Here are a few things to keep in mind:

1. Appreciation isn't just a "soft" concept. It has a highly beneficial effect on your body.

2. Appreciation, which is often easier to activate than other core heart feelings, can shift your attitudes and perceptions quickly.

3. Appreciation helps draw additional fulfilling situations toward you. What you send out does come back.

4. Find something to appreciate when things aren't going your way, not just when it's convenient.

5. Make a conscious effort to look for things in your life that you can appreciate, and try to remember them. Writing up an occasional appreciation list will help.

6. Stay on the lookout for areas in your life where you've adapted and are taking things for granted. Try to find new appreciation in these areas.

Someone like Papa John was probably blessed from the start with an ability to appreciate. He made appreciation look easy, but no doubt even he had to work at it from time to time. It's the challenges in life that force us to mature and reach our full potential. Appreciate them!

## Power Tool 2: Nonjudgment

It seems as if people live in a sea of judgment. The mind likes to separate, categorize, and catalog information. It sizes up everything and everybody in order to reach understanding. Unfortunately, as we've said before, knowledge isn't understanding.

An active mind without heart direction tends to adopt strong opinions about much of what it takes in. These often-rigid mind-sets provide a basis for deciding what we like or don't like, who's right and who's not, what's good and what's bad.

In the process, we become highly skilled at making judgments. In many ways, this ability is priceless. Judgments allow us to make personal choices. Without judgments, we'd never be able to decide which car to purchase or what food to select at the grocery store. As we grow and mature into adulthood, many of our judgments become more refined. For example, we come to know the difference between someone who's telling us the truth about his or her product and someone who's just trying to sell us something. Our refined judgment helps us see that distinction.

When judgment is used to help us make personal choices or solid business decisions, it's a positive thing. But judgment can be misused. When we speak negatively of judgment here, we're talking about those rigid, negative opinions that separate us from others—that let us point the finger and consider ourselves superior. Judgments can be made about almost anything, including issues, places, things, and (especially) people. More times than not, such judgments are based on incomplete, often prejudicial information.

Can you think of anyone who's close to you now whom you didn't like when you first met? Someone about whom you made a high-speed judgment, deciding that he just wasn't the kind of person that appealed to you? Sometimes people end up happily married to that person they judged. Their first opinion seems humorous in light of their current feelings.

When we judge so easily about so many different things, we have to wonder how much understanding and new intelligence these judgments are blocking out.

### Developing Heart-Based Discrimination

True heart-based discrimination is very different from head-based judgment. The latter, by far the more common, is often rationalized into virtue: "I wasn't really *judging* my boss; I was just *assessing* him." But how often is that true? While genuine assessment is energy-efficient and beneficial, assessment too often provides a convenient smokescreen for judgment. Without enough heart mixed into your discrimination, your assessments become colored with a wide variety of assumptions that lead to judgmental thoughts, feelings, and perspectives.

One way to know if you're assessing from the heart or the head is to see how neutral you are about your opinions. While the head stands firm, the heart allows new understanding to become available. The heart doesn't shut the door on information or insight; in fact, it gives you the awareness needed to become more neutral, letting things unfold.

Nonjudgment is generous and allowing. Nonjudgmental perceptions aren't overattached to or overidentified with what's wrong. Thus becoming more neutral is the first step toward nonjudgment. Eventually, as you take further steps, you begin to see the deeper aspects of life and people—aspects that are so wonderful that some might call them divine. Instead of quickly identifying people's faults and seeing their character through that fault-finding lens, you begin to lead with love. Not only do the people around you start to look better, but your entire spirit is enhanced by that generous, life-giving quality.

When your heart is on-line, you have less tendency to focus on the negative things in life. That doesn't mean you like or agree with everything you see; that's not the point. But your own measuring, confining opinions lose their vice grip on you. When you evaluate with the heart, you can still have opinions, but you have other choices as well—feelings of compassion and appreciation that may not have been there before. In time, the warmth of those feelings will begin to appeal to you so much more than your judgments and opinions that you'll have the motivation to set those mental constructs aside.

When you're run by the head, making assessments and judgments seems like the most important thing. You base all your values and decisions on those conclusions. We're not saying that evaluating issues or people rationally is wrong. But evaluations that lack the heart can't possibly show you the whole picture.

Heart-based discrimination keeps wholeness in mind. As a natural result, it allows you to invest less energy in the judgments and opinions you've formed. Once you've learned to lead with the heart, you'll still be aware of those opinions, of course. But you'll also always be open to new options; your heart and mind won't be closed or constricted.

Negative judgments simply aren't healthy. Like other deficits, they create stress and incoherence in your biological systems. All those negative attitudes and feelings running through your body are toxic, and they shut off the riches of the heart. And there's a further downside of judgment: because of the negative impact on our bodies, the person who judges is the one who's hurt the most. You could almost say that our systems are designed to even the score.

Say a driver pulls out in front of you, blocking the intersection and causing you to miss the light. This makes you furious, because you were running late anyway. You start to write a mental book of judgment on people like him—rude drivers and so on. He drives off happily, never knowing what you think of him;

you, on the other hand, are riddled with judgmental energy that's depleting, draining, and imbalancing your system as it courses through your veins.

It takes a lot of energy to adopt and sustain judgments—to scan your surroundings, notice faults, assess their significance, and hold on to and defend opinions. Add in the emotional energy used to fuel judgments, and the inefficient investment increases dramatically.

It's impossible to know all sides of most issues—or know all aspects of a person's character or motivation—so why expend all of that energy judging? Don't we have better things to do? Yes—but judgment feels satisfying because it's a way of defending our own position.

At a military installation in Texas a few years ago, I (Howard) was doing a program for about seventy-five drug and alcohol counselors. The group was made up of uniformed personnel as well as civilian employees.

The program was going well, but I noticed that a man sitting in the back, a civilian, wasn't participating. He stared at me intensely, so he was obviously listening, but he didn't open his guidebook or do any of the written exercises with the group.

Initially I decided that he was probably just one of those tough guys. Maybe a former military man; yes, probably a drill sergeant. I could imagine that he'd been forced to attend by his supervisor and that, not liking all this "heart stuff," he'd come with an attitude.

By the time we took a break, my judgments had convinced me that it was even worse than that. This guy was probably always a discipline problem who gave his supervisors no end of grief.

At the break, the major in charge of the division asked me how I thought it was going. "Fine," I said, "but there's this one guy who's not participating. He just sits there like a bump on a log and hasn't even opened his guidebook."

"Who is it?" the officer asked.

When I pointed him out, the major chuckled. "That's Robert," he said. "He's one of our very best counselors. He doesn't look it, but he's legally blind. He doesn't open the guidebook because he can't read it."

Humbled by my own judgments and by how ridiculously far they'd led me astray, I made a point of speaking to Robert. Instead of giving me the attitude that I'd thought was written all over his face, he said that this was one of the most powerful seminars he'd ever taken and he wished everyone on the base could take it.

Remember, the mind likes to assume it "knows what it knows," but often its perceptions are just not accurate. Yet strong judgments are made all the time— every day, every hour—based on limited information. Think of the judgments we make based only on what someone else has said or on something we read or saw on TV. When we judge someone and then adopt an attitude toward that person, we're shutting down other possibilities and locking ourselves away from the insight of our hearts.

At some point in our evolution, that might've been the best we could do. It's conceivable that primitive man, totally out of control of his emotions and without much cognitive development, made judgments that saved his life. They cost him a lot, but if that's what it took to remind him to avoid saber-toothed tigers or sticking his hand in a fire, so be it.

As you're reading this, some of you may be saying, "I need my judgments to survive, to tell me what to avoid or embrace in the world." We hear you—but what we're saying is that mind-based judging is a costly, even primitive, approach. We're standing at the threshold of new possibilities in our evolution. A better, more efficient choice is heart-based discrimination. You're capable of it. Why not give it a try?

### Avoiding Self-Judgment

Even more detrimental are our *self*-judgments. When we don't meet our own standards, we're often harder on ourselves than we would be on others. Just as I (Howard) formed my presumptions about Robert, we can easily form mistaken opinions about ourselves and even our own motives.

Few of us grew up in optimally supportive home environments. The opinions others had about us in those formative years sometimes ring in our heads for decades. If our early caregivers judged us harshly or unfairly, we may continue to take those judgments about ourselves at face value instead of keeping a loving, open attitude toward ourselves.

Making a mistake and then judging ourselves harshly is like paying compound interest on a bad investment. We don't always act in ways that please us, but beating ourselves up over mistakes doesn't do any good.

By developing new heart intelligence, you can objectively look at your mistakes and learn from them without going into judgment and recrimination. You can give yourself the support and encouragement you would automatically give to someone you love. It's not always easy to do, but it's well worth the effort.

Because judging and self-judging happen so mechanically, we can easily immerse ourselves in judgmental perceptions and attitudes without realizing that we're doing it. After all, everyone around us at the office or in the family is doing judging too. We're socially conditioned to endlessly judge.

One of the classic illustrations of judgmentalism is so contradictory that it's almost funny. It centers on something that often happens after self-improvement seminars at which we've had some breakthroughs and new insights. We go home and our success goes right to our heads. It's called the I'm-more-developed-than-you-are game. Instead of appreciating our own growth, we start pointing the finger at everybody else who doesn't know what we know. We've all done it.

So here's a cue to be on the lookout for that tendency even while reading this book. We've drawn your attention to certain energy drains. As you become more aware of them in yourself, it's natural to become more aware of them in the world around you. If you're not careful, you'll find yourself thinking, "How little appreciation she has!" or "I used to be like that, but now I'm more emotionally mature." Before you know it, you'll be making judgments about other people's judgments! "Look how he made up his mind so quickly. What a judgmental person."

This is fair warning: if we indulge in these kinds of self-righteous judgments, we'll undermine the gains we're making in other areas of heart cultivation. Don't fall for the temptation. Why short-circuit yourself? Turn your new awareness about energy drains and the power of the heart toward yourself. Focus on your own growth with love. As you become more loving with yourself, that generosity will spread to others as well.

Of course, your head is still going to assess and have opinions. That's necessary for decision-making, as we've said. However, it's possible to create that ultimate partnership between heart and head to guide your decisions toward what's best for the whole. But you can't experience the more refined aspects of heart discernment without reducing the inner static and noise created by judgment.

We're not going to eliminate all judgmentalism overnight. It's done step by step, through increasing ratios of catching ourselves. The first step in that process is to notice your judgmental and self-judgmental tendencies. See if these tendencies apply to you:

*Judgmental Tendencies*

1. I am quick to criticize.
2. I have a tendency to notice lots of things that bother me.
3. I have many strong opinions, especially about what's wrong with the world.
4. I feel that I'm right about most things and other people are usually wrong.
5. I experience me-against-them thoughts and feelings regularly.

*Self-Judgmental Tendencies*

1. I'm always criticizing myself.
2. I can never do anything right.
3. I feel that everyone does things better than I do.

If you feel that you're judging too much, don't worry. You're far from alone. Remember that we live in a sea of judgment and judgmental patterning; the world around us reinforces this kind of behavior. Because we've become socially entrained to judgmental patterns, it takes some practice to get beyond them.

You have to eliminate judgment in stages, reducing the amount of energy you spend judging a step at a time. You will, of course, notice things that you don't agree with and form opinions about what you perceive. You can't get around that. But as you practice nonjudgment, you can reduce the impact of your judgments and their detrimental effects.

### Practicing Nonjudgment

It's easy to have one or two unsavory, judgmental thoughts about someone, but that's not usually where we stop. We typically move on to more and more judgmental thoughts; and then we emotionally react to those thoughts, reinforcing the energy-draining practice and locking it into our mental and emotional circuitry.

Here's an exercise that will help change this pattern. When you start to have thoughts that are judgmental, sound the alarm. Then, as soon as you catch yourself, watch the next thought and the next thought and the next; stop the judgment before it goes any further. Sometimes it takes going to a deep neutral to stop the momentum. FREEZE-FRAME and hold to neutral and see what happens.

For example, suppose you're walking down a deserted street alone at night. At the end of the block, you see four tough-looking guys standing around drinking. You might say, "These guys look like trouble. I think I'll go down another street—one with better lighting." Now turning down another street might be a good idea—even a lifesaving idea—but if you add emotional energy to your perception of the men, it turns into a judgment.

You have to admit that you don't really know who these people are or what they're doing. You might as well be saying, "These guys are low-life scum, worthless human beings." And while you're stirring up judgmental toxins in your system, it feels quite natural to move on to blame: "Where are the cops when you need them? What's our society come to, allowing bums like this to run loose on the street?" If your fear kicks in as well, it's only icing on the cake.

So coming across those guys on the corner really did cause you harm — not from them, but from yourself. You didn't have to think and feel those things. You could have stopped yourself from causing such a toxic effect by going to the heart to keep your perspective balanced and poised — even if you chose to change your route.

Heart discrimination would at least have gotten you to neutral: "I don't know who these guys are, but I think I'll turn down another street just in case. Why walk into a potentially dangerous situation?"

The way to eliminate judgment is to make a more conscious effort to surrender mind to heart and find a solid neutral. You don't have to buy into anything or see anything in an idealistic light. But from a neutral place you can at least say, "What if . . ." What if the situation isn't the way you think it is, or what if it *is?* By not forming opinions or making hasty assumptions, you leave yourself open to the truth. From that place of neutral nonjudgment, your heart can come on-line and you can watch your perceptions shift.

Once you're in neutral and your heart is engaged, activate your appreciation for life and consciously generate compassion and care as you decide your next move. This practice alone will eliminate a huge percentage of your judgments.

It's the mind, when not connected to the heart, that feels the need to pigeonhole everything and cut people, places, and issues down to size. When you're perceiving from the heart, you won't see so much to dislike and it won't feel right to be so judgmental. Heart intelligence changes the circuitry on mechanical, judgmental patterns.

When you find yourself in strong judgment, use the FREEZE-FRAME technique to help you get to neutral and find a more balanced, intuitive perspective. Ask your heart to help you get out of judgment. Then activate the power tool of appreciation. Try to find something to appreciate about the person, place, or issue you're judging.

Using these tools to stop payment on judgments is an act of self-care. Religions talk about nonjudgment, but only saints seem to know how to pull it off. The core heart feeling of nonjudgment is a state of balanced neutral. Armed with the science and the cybernetics behind nonjudgment, anyone can do it. Nonjudgment is really the next step for human survival and evolution. Use your heart intelligence to actualize the nonjudgment that you know is possible, and release yourself.

## Power Tool 3: Forgiveness

As you begin to practice the heart power tools, an interesting thing happens. You may find yourself doing well in many areas—discovering the advantages of living a heart-directed life, learning about the power of love, and beginning to sincerely appreciate more of the world around you. Because you're starting to add love to your life, the textures of experience feel richer, more engaging. You're increasingly more likely to recognize tension when you feel it. You're getting better at cutting off stress at the pass. If you're starting to feel proud of yourself for these improvements, you should be. These changes alone will dramatically increase the quality of your life. And they'll continue to deepen and grow. You're definitely on the right track.

But experience has shown us that as people faithfully strive to rid themselves of the mental and emotional patterns that create incoherence, they eventually come face to face with some of their toughest issues.

Learning how to get to neutral quickly when someone cuts you off in traffic is great. Managing your anxiety over confrontation at the office by feeling sincere appreciation for something is invaluable. But what about those old issues that sit in your deficit pile for years and are still draining your quality of life? Times that you were mistreated. Times that the other person knew—or should have known—that what she did would hurt you, and she did it anyway. Times that your love or trust was betrayed. Times that someone else wronged the one you love.

Forgiveness is one of the trickiest power tools there is. People often say they've forgiven someone for something, then go on to suffer from incoherence for weeks, months, even years. Betrayal, injustice, insults, and slights not only cause us pain, they insult our pride. They feel intensely personal, and it's hard to let them go. So putting those old, lingering wounds to rest requires a stronger act of forgiveness.

As difficult as it seems, you can be sure of this: at the core of the heart, you have the power to move beyond the old issues that are still hindering your freedom. The hardest things—the ones that push you up against your limits—are the very things you need to address to make a quantum leap into a fresh inner and outer life.

### Loving Your Way Through It

Forgiveness for the big things takes time. This is an area where you may need to build up a little heart power first. Use the HeartMath Solution tools and techniques to eliminate as many other deficits and energy leaks as you can. Then use your heart intelligence to think, feel, and act in ways that you know accumulate assets by adding to your store of core heart feeling experiences.

By eliminating deficits while gaining assets, you'll increase your inner energy reserves, gaining substantially more power to love and forgive. Be patient with yourself, but keep going for it. If you make consistent, heart-directed efforts to let go of the past, over time you'll dissolve old, unresolved feelings and reach a more complete state of forgiveness.

New understanding will come to you even as you *try* to forgive. Through heart discrimination, you may realize that the people you feel resentment for might have been doing the best they could at the time they did you wrong. For whatever reason, maybe they just couldn't help their wrongdoing. That possibility is worth considering.

Look at it this way. There are probably times that you've done something that somebody else had trouble forgiving. Whatever it was—big or small—someone didn't like it and resented you for it.

For all you know, that person could be reading this same book (or another book about forgiveness), scanning his past to see who and what he needs to forgive. And you could come to mind, perhaps even topping the list.

If you knew that this person was harboring a grudge, you'd most likely hope for understanding and forgiveness. Maybe you're not proud of your behavior either, but there were compelling factors that influenced you at the time. Maybe you were doing the best you knew under the circumstances, though that doesn't *excuse* your behavior. See if you can offer that same latitude to the people you need to forgive. Try to see things more neutrally—that is, without emotional prejudice—to reach a deeper understanding.

Even as you read this, though, doesn't a certain person come to mind who doesn't *deserve* to be forgiven, who ought to be an exception to the offer of latitude? We've all encountered people who've acted in a consciously malicious manner, or who've been habitually abusive or reckless—and have hurt us in the process. We're by no means suggesting that you hang around and take the hurt. If someone can't be trusted, know that. Then get out of harm's way.

But in the long run, it's not a question of whether someone *deserves* to be forgiven. You're not forgiving your transgressor for his or her sake; you're doing it for yourself. Forgiveness is simply the most energy-efficient option you face, and the only one that will foster health and well-being. It frees you from the toxic, debilitating drain of holding a grudge. Don't let villains live rent-free in your head. If they've hurt you in the past, why let them keep hurting you year after year in your mind? It's not worth it—but it takes heart effort to stop it. You can muster the heart power to forgive those who've wronged you as a way of looking out for yourself. It's one thing you can be totally selfish about.

Take it slowly. The deepest resentments are wrapped up in a lot of hurt and pain. We think we're protecting ourselves by not forgiving. Acknowledge that and go easy on yourself. Forgiveness means that you've decided not to let the pain keep festering inside, even if it comes up only once in awhile. Forgiveness is a powerful yet challenging tool that will support and honor you, even in the most extreme circumstances.

### Using Heart Power—The Real Thing

David McArthur, one of our colleagues here at HeartMath, used to be an assistant attorney general in New Mexico. Years ago, he and his wife volunteered to take in a distant cousin who, as it turned out, had serious mental and emotional problems. After living with them for several months, the cousin pulled out a gun and killed David's wife for no apparent reason.

Despite his grief and pain—and that of his one-year-old daughter—David was somehow able to gradually understand that this young man couldn't be held accountable for his actions. Realizing that the man was incapable of reason, David forgave him.

The crime was so horrible that the residents of his New Mexico town were up in arms. Out of his compassion for this disturbed young man, David found a lawyer to take his case and fought to have the young man committed to a mental institution instead of standing trial for first-degree murder.

David's act of forgiveness was extraordinary. It would have been perfectly understandable for him to have carried a rage toward his wife's murderer to his grave. He could easily have turned against himself for his decision to take the boy in or condemned the injustice of God and the universe for betraying his kindness. Instead, he found enough power in his heart to forgive this young man and move on with his life. He even visited the cousin in prison and told him—with complete sincerity—that he forgave him. He showed remarkable strength and maturity of heart.

David claims, "The first thing you have to do to forgive is to send love to yourself to heal the hurt and pain you feel. As that pain is transformed, it gives you the power and ability to love and forgive others."

David didn't have the HeartMath Solution tools and techniques at the time, but fortunately he was a man with a big heart. For most people, overcoming the justifiably negative thoughts and feelings associated with something so horrible would take a lot of work. That's where FREEZE-FRAME comes in, providing the ability to see things more clearly. Activating appreciation and nonjudgment as best you can also helps significantly with forgiveness. As you seek to clear out the emotional residue associated with a major crisis, the regular practice of CUT-THRU and HEART LOCK-IN (two techniques you'll learn about later) is invaluable. Through the use of all of these tools and techniques, you can come into deeper contact with your heart intelligence, which leads to greater love. It takes all these skills for most of us to find the power of forgiveness when we face a highly challenging situation like David's.

Forgiveness of this degree takes a lot of heart power. To generate that power, the best way to go is love. Ultimately, the one thing—the only thing—that can dissolve old resentments and hurts is love, the mother of all the heart power tools. Approach forgiveness by increasing the power of love you send to yourself, and then apply that love to forgiveness. The rewards for taking on such deep work certainly outweigh the distress of continuing to live with the hurts and pains.

As you make the effort, you'll discover that forgiveness often involves many negative emotional conditions—a jumble of justification, blame, hurt, a sense of unfairness, overcare, and judgment all rolled into one. All of these feelings can glom on to whatever someone or something did (or didn't do) to you and make the issue all but impenetrable.

The incoherence that results from holding on to resentments and unforgiving attitudes keeps you from being aligned with your true self and blocks you from your next level of quality life experience. Metaphorically, it's the curtain hanging between the room you're living in now and a new room—much larger and full of beautiful objects. The act of forgiveness removes the curtain. In fact, clearing up your old accounts can free up so much energy that you jump right into a whole new house. Forgiving releases you from the punishment of a self-made prison in which you're both the inmate and the jailer.

### Forgiving Yourself

Above all, don't hesitate to turn the power of your love inward if you need to. As hard as it is to forgive someone else, it's sometimes much harder to forgive ourselves. When a loved one dies, we think, "If only I'd come home sooner, or had taken different action, or had told him one more thing." It's as if we're somehow the guilty party in their death. When we lose a job or a relationship, we may start by blaming others, but we generally end up pointing the finger at ourselves: "I should have been different." In some people, this tendency is so strong that a monologue of self-blame runs in their heads all the time. They're blessed with an inner critic who always gives their decisions and actions bad reviews.

In the popular movie *Good Will Hunting*, the main character, Will, a young genius, experienced a host of emotional problems and was headed for a life of crime and jail time. Because he couldn't move beyond his problems, he was squandering his genius.

A friendly mentor who cared took him to several psychiatrists for help, but they couldn't make a dent. He was too smart for them. Finally, after much work, a psychologist with a big heart did get through.

Because Will had been abused as a child, he carried a tremendous burden of hurt and anger. A child who looks for love and is met with abuse and hostility feels unlovable. He blames himself, even though it's clearly not his fault.

When Will's psychologist helped him reach a point of self-forgiveness — when Will realized at a *feeling* level, not a *conceptual* level, that the past wasn't his fault — he experienced a dramatic breakthrough. All of the pieces in the puzzle of his life fell into place, and his genius started to manifest with purpose and balance. In the last scene, he drives off on the open highway, freed from the past and headed toward a new life and love. When he finally made contact with his deeper heart, everything shifted. True forgiveness can change your life; but, as Will learned, you have to apply it first and foremost to yourself. Otherwise, your guilt and self-blame will block the free flow of energy.

Take a moment now and ask yourself if you're holding any grudges against yourself. Whatever they might be, find a way to forgive them. Forgiving another person is going only halfway, if you keep part of the blame for yourself.

### Watching Out for Compromised Forgiveness

The secret to mastering forgiveness is learning how to do it *all the way*. It's easy to apply half a cup of forgiveness to a three-gallon problem. While you can appreciate the fact that you made the effort, that "compromised forgiveness" won't really do the job.

Suppose you're the office manager of a corporation. You enjoy your job overseeing the support staff and always strive to be fair. One day, as you're passing the coffee room, you overhear a particular secretary gossiping about you. She says a few things that are really insulting. You confront her immediately, but you're still steamed.

It takes some work to find a place in your heart for forgiveness. After working on it gently over the next few days, you finally get there. It's worth the effort.

The cloud that had been looming over you, dampening your energy, seems to lift. You feel like yourself again.

Then comes the time to recommend the secretaries for raises, and you start to pass her by—not because of her work, but because of what she said about you. Apparently your forgiveness wasn't complete. You eye with relish the chance to get her. But if you take that chance, you'll pay for it out of your own energy reserves.

Be on the lookout for compromised forgiveness. You'll notice it any time you make a statement that qualifies how much you've forgiven: "I've forgiven her, but . . ." The words vary, but the theme's the same: "I've forgiven him for cheating on me, but not for betraying me with my best friend." Or "I've forgiven her, but I never want to speak to her or see her again." Compromised forgiveness leaves you *believing* that you've forgiven someone. Then you discover, even years later, that the mere mention of his name still causes an uncomfortable sensation.

Your initial effort was worthy—just not thorough enough to bring release at the cellular level. It may be that you actually *did* forgive that person for everything you knew about at the time, but over the years other aspects have come to the surface. Uprooting resentment is a lot like pulling out a thorn. Even if you get most of it out, a little bit of the tip can stay in. That final bit has to work itself out later. And when it does, you'll discover that there's more to forgive.

Compromised forgiveness means that somewhere, somehow or another, the effort was incomplete. That lack of completion can mean the difference between a breakthrough into a completely new and different life experience and the same old patterns repeating themselves. Without completion, it's hard for the gifts of true forgiveness to be bestowed.

### Blunting the Razor's Edge

Once you get past all of the justifications and make solid heart contact, forgiveness gets easier and release comes quickly.

As a young man just out of school, I (Howard) worked in a retail store at a mall. One day a wealthy Japanese woman—a regular customer—came in and offered me another job. She was opening a new store that would sell fine imported Japanese china and art objects. She wanted me to manage it for her and offered me substantially more money than I was making at the time. I decided to give it a try. I left my other job and began helping her set up this new business.

During the first week, she had me pick her up at her house and drive her around while she picked out displays, carpeting, and so forth. A week into the job, I was ten minutes late picking her up. She admonished me sternly for my tardiness.

Being a bit spirited (or, to say it more honestly, a bit emotionally reactive), I delivered—with some passion—numerous valid excuses for being late and reasons why she shouldn't talk to me so sternly.

The rest of the day I served her politely and efficiently. Everything seemed fine. When I got home that night, I checked my answering machine and found a message from her saying that I'd been fired for disrespect. I was shocked and enraged. The next morning I called my old boss and asked for my job back, but he'd already replaced me. I was now unemployed.

That night I got together with some of my friends, including Doc. I told them what had happened and how I'd been screwed. They concurred that it seemed a bit unfair: the woman had pulled the trigger a little too quickly, and yes, I was in a tough spot. As I continued to feel sorry for myself about the situation, some of the guys, being the good friends that they were, began to offer a more sobering view of the situation.

"You know, Razor, you've got an awfully sharp edge too," they reminded me. That was, after all, the reason I'd gotten the nickname in the first place—mental sharpness and emotional impulsiveness combined. Their comments were lighthearted but honest.

I (Doc) remember this incident well. I could see that Howard was having a hard time with his situation. I knew that once resentment and self-pity kicked in, they'd be hard to shake loose; and I knew that the whole situation had wounded Howard's pride. So I made a few suggestions. "Don't do the obvious thing. Do what most other people wouldn't do. Clean up any mess you've left behind. Whether you feel like it or not, go ahead and forgive this woman. That will put this incident to rest and free you from weeks or months of resentment." It was a tall order for a young man who felt insulted, but I knew the depth of Howard's sincerity. If he wrestled with himself and got in touch with his heart, I knew he could do it.

As soon as I (Howard) heard Doc's advice, I sensed that he was right. After I'd pondered it in my heart awhile, I realized that forgiveness was in order. The next morning I decided to drive over to the woman's house and apologize as a way of demonstrating my forgiveness.

On the way, however, I started to feel that my plan was stupid. I didn't need to go through with this. Again—and with fresh pain—I felt that she'd been too quick to admonish me for my lateness, had unfairly fired me and left me in a mess! The more I thought about it, the more I didn't want to forgive her, much less apologize in person. The head was compromising my true heart's intentions.

I finally stopped the car in a wooded area and went to my heart for direction. I sat there for a few minutes and sought a better understanding of the woman and the possible reasons she might have had for firing me. Able now to put myself in her place, I realized that she too was in a bad position, having no manager for her new store. Perhaps I really *did* need to forgive her, whether I thought what she'd done had been right or not. I knew that I'd played a part in the outcome; it wasn't just her. The journey continued.

As I got to her street, my mind and emotions started to get the best of me again. Thoughts like, "If I do this right, maybe she'll at least have pity and give me some severance pay," crept in. Next it was thoughts like, "I'll do it just to prove I can, but it's still not quite fair." My mind was getting even slicker, making its last stand. "Forgiveness with a hidden agenda to get something instead of giving. What a concept."

I again stopped the car, realizing that this act of forgiveness had to be sincere—with no hidden agenda; otherwise, nothing would be accomplished. Unless my forgiveness was genuine and from the heart, all I'd have is a great story to tell my friends. No real release would come for me or her. With that understanding, I went deeper and mustered as much sincerity as I could.

By now I was getting tired of this game. I knew that I needed to just grow up and forgive and apologize as best I could. I rang her doorbell and focused in my heart as I waited. Looking a bit surprised and even offended that I'd dared show up at her house, she held the door open just a crack. Her demeanor toward me had all the warmth of a meat locker.

Deep in my heart, and now finally undeterred, I told her that I was sorry and that I understood how hard it could be for people to deal with my reactiveness. I said sincerely that I had no hard feelings, that I hoped I'd caused her no harm and wished her the very best with the new store. In a monotone, she said thank you and closed the door.

The drive home was a lot smoother than the one to her house. Although she'd given me no obvious confirmation or release, I didn't need it, because I knew I'd come clean with her from the heart. I hadn't compromised.

If you're waiting for the happy ending, here it is: I freed up my energy and learned an invaluable lesson. I knew that it would now be much easier to forgive in the future. And I had new appreciation for my friends and for their honest advice, which had helped me gain so much from the experience. Going deep in the heart to find forgiveness had opened new doors for me.

## Amping Up Your Heart's Power

We've introduced only three potential power tools of the heart in this chapter—appreciation, nonjudgment, and forgiveness. There are many others. Every core heart feeling is a potential power tool—compassion, patience, courage, and others. Part of your own development will involve finding the ones you need to cultivate in yourself. With sincerity and coherence behind them, these tools will help you build the power for transformation that lies waiting within you.

A friend of ours, Jim Cathcart, talks about how people grow into their full potential in his book *The Acorn Principle*. Jim believes that fulfillment is based on two elements, awareness and performance. He says, "Self-development comes from the increased awareness of where you are right now and learning what is needed in order to grow. And self-expression is how you perform, what you do about it." [1]

It may take time to develop your core heart potential, but as you uncover a deeper connection with the power of the heart, you'll find more appreciation, love, and forgiveness at its core. New freedom will come as you clean out old mind-sets, hurts, pains, and resistances.

The HeartMath Solution power tools offer ways to gain direct access to your own heart's power. That power removes incoherence. With less static and discord in your system, your highest intelligence, your true spirit, has the chance to enter your day-to-day world, and more fulfillment will be your just reward.

## KEY POINTS TO REMEMBER

➤ Sincerity is the generator that brings core heart feelings such as appreciation and forgiveness into coherence and gives them power.

➤ Opening your heart is like putting a wide-angle lens on the camera of your perception. Suddenly, more of the world comes into view.

➤ When you have a major insight about something you want to change, you run the risk of losing your initial passion (and thus your impetus to change). By rekindling appreciation, you can restore the initial excitement you had about your insight.

➤ Judgments create stress and incoherence, and these limit the full range of our intelligence. Yet we're socially conditioned to judge.

➤ One of the important things to note about the downside of judgment is that the person judging is the one who's hurt the most.

➤ Making a mistake and then judging yourself harshly is like paying compound interest on a bad investment.

➤ The heart can give you the awareness needed to become more neutral, letting things unfold. That's what nonjudgment is all about.

➤ When you find yourself in strong judgment, use the FREEZE-FRAME technique to get to neutral and find a more balanced, intuitive perspective.

➤ Armed with the science and the cybernetics behind nonjudgment, anyone can do it. Nonjudgment is an important next step in human survival and evolution.

➤ Uprooting resentment is a lot like pulling out a thorn. Even if you get most of it out, a little bit of the tip can stay in and rankle.

➤ Compromised forgiveness means that somewhere, somehow or another, the effort was incomplete. That lack of completion can mean the difference between a breakthrough into a completely new and different life experience and the same old patterns repeating themselves.

PART 3

# Advanced Heart Intelligence

Parts I and II of *The HeartMath Solution* provided a solid understanding of heart intelligence and the tools needed to access it. The FREEZE-FRAME technique, the asset/deficit balance sheet, and the heart power tools introduced in those parts give you practical, hands-on ways to unfold your heart intelligence and use it in daily life. But there's more to be gained from the heart.

Part III will focus on the next, more refined level of this system—managing emotions and increasing your connection to heart intelligence.

Because emotions are very complex, they can be hard to manage. It's essential, however, to harness the power of emotions in order to increase and maintain internal coherence. We'll present an in-depth view of emotions, providing an understanding of how they work and explaining how emotional management is often both neglected and compromised.

Part III also includes a chapter on a fourth heart power tool, care—and its counterpart, overcare. Overcare is often at the core of emotional problems. Once identified, it can be eliminated; that step allows a new level of emotional management to be attained.

Two advanced techniques are introduced in this section, CUT-THRU and HEART LOCK-IN. CUT-THRU is a technique that uses the power of the heart to bring your emotions into balance and erase emotional blocks from the past.

HEART LOCK-IN provides an experience of sustained contact with your heart intelligence. As you become accustomed to this rich connection, you'll gain new intuitive and creative insights. HEART LOCK-IN is also used to bring the body into a more coherent, revitalized state.

In Part III you will:

➤ Understand emotions and emotional management

➤ Learn to distinguish between care and overcare

➤ Learn and apply the CUT-THRU technique for greater emotional management

➤ Learn and apply the HEART LOCK-IN technique to expand and refine access to heart intelligence

# CHAPTER 7

# Understanding the Mystery of Emotions

Toni Roberts first started to experience feelings of depression when she was a young girl. She remembers feeling sad all the time, wanting to stay in her room and not play with other children. As she went into her teen years, it got worse. Daily bouts of crying were normal for her. To those around her, though, she appeared to be on top of the world. She was a good student and a well-liked leader. But Toni participated in leadership roles and school activities such as cheerleading as a diversion, an attempt to compensate for the pain and emptiness she felt on the inside.

Her depression continued on into her thirties as she struggled to raise her family and manage her successful career as a professional fundraiser.

Toni knew she had a serious problem, and she desperately wanted help. She tried everything from religion and prayer to meditation, therapy, and anti-depressants but found only random, temporary relief. After decades of trying to rid herself of this emotional disease, she finally came to the stark conclusion that she would *never* feel better. All she could expect to experience was feelings of hopelessness.

One day a friend told Toni about HeartMath. She was tired of chasing a cure for her problem but decided to attend a HeartMath training program anyway. During the weekend she made a sincere effort to make contact with her heart, and during one of the many exercises something remarkable happened. She had a breakthrough, a profound experience of hope and release. For days after the seminar she felt different—better—but how could this be?

Toni had had temporary breakthroughs before but they'd never lasted. She feared now that she'd slip back into the depths of chronic depression. After so many years it was hard to accept that by going to her heart she could be free of it. Toni kept practicing what she'd learned, however, using FREEZE-FRAME when she felt the need, consciously activating core heart feelings, and doing HEART LOCK INS. Within a month, the fear that her depression would come back was gone. She knew that her emotional problems were behind her. They seemed now like nothing more than a bad dream. As her health continued to improve dramatically, a joyfulness, a lightness, and a zest for life replaced her depression. That was six years ago. Toni now works for HeartMath and says that her life continues to become more fulfilling and enriched every day.

Toni's rather dramatic experience is a wonderful example of what can happen when our hearts come alive. Emotional problems are among the most difficult to deal with, especially if they're long-standing, as Toni's were. Perhaps Tony had even looked to her heart for help before, but because she didn't know how to activate heart intelligence with consistency, she continued to suffer for years. Once she *did* make that deeper heart connection, however, her emotions responded accordingly and her life took a major turn for the better.

## Emotions

What would it be like if you somehow managed to climb to the top of Mount Everest but couldn't feel the exhilarating rush of excitement? What if you spent time with family or close friends but couldn't feel the love between you? Our emotions are such a natural part of our existence that we take them for granted. They allow us to experience the textures and colors of life. Without them, we can still climb Mount Everest and spend time with our family and friends, but what's the point? Emotions—and emotions alone—give meaning to our lives.

The ability to laugh or cry, to feel alternately pensive and blissful, imbues our existence with beauty and value. We crave feeling, because the experience of emotion makes life matter. It transforms our world from an objective, conceptual fact into a living, breathing experience.

Facts are crucial too, but in a pinch the compelling power of emotion almost always wins out. As the English writer Thomas Browne said in 1690, "Men live by intervals of reason under the sovereignty of humor and passion." With a force of their own that must be honored and appreciated, emotions consistently transcend reason in our lives. And yet they remain a great mystery.

While the enigmatic power of emotions can enrich our lives beyond measure, it can destroy us just as easily. Emotion, not reason, is the force behind a large majority of the wars and conflicts the world has seen. The intelligence needed to manage this potent inner force, using it for our highest good, has eluded mankind for centuries.

The emotional frontier is truly the next frontier to conquer in human understanding. The opportunity we face now, even before that frontier is fully explored and settled, is to develop our emotional potential and accelerate rather dramatically into a new state of being.

The word "emotion" literally means "energy in motion." It's derived from the Latin verb meaning "to move." While a feeling—a closely related concept—is any conscious experience of sensation, an emotion is a *strong* feeling, a feeling such as love, joy, sorrow, or anger that *moves* us. An emotion generates various complex reactions with both mental and physiological changes and accompanying autonomic nervous system manifestations. [1] What we think of as emotion is the experience of energy moving through our bodies. In itself, emotional energy is neutral. It's the feeling sensation and physiological reaction that make a specific emotion positive or negative, and it's our thoughts about it that give it meaning.

Emotions serve as carrier waves for the entire spectrum of feelings. When our hearts are in a state of coherence, we more easily experience feelings such as love, care, appreciation, and kindness. On the other hand, feelings such as irritation, anger, hurt, and envy are more likely to occur when the head and heart are out of alignment. Our emotional experiences become imprinted in our brain cells and memory, where they form patterns that influence our behavior. [2]

## Feeling Is Faster Than Thought

E motional energy works at a higher speed than thought. This is because the feeling world operates at a higher speed than the mind. Scientists have repeatedly confirmed that our emotional reactions show up in brain activity before we even have time to think. We evaluate everything emotionally *as we perceive it*. We think about it *afterwards*. [3]

If emotional energy works faster than the mind, how can we expect to manage our emotions with our thoughts? Good question. And in fact it takes *more* than the mind to manage emotions. The heart's coherent power is required as well. Heart coherence helps balance our emotional state. It aligns head and heart to facilitate higher brain function, which appears to create a direct link to intuition or super-high-speed intelligence. Intuition bypasses mental analysis and gives us direct perception independent of any reasoning process. [4]

Intuition gives us clarity on how to direct and manage our feelings before we invest emotional energy in them.

Emotions in themselves aren't really intelligent. But anything that has a flow   as emotion and thought do—has a theme of intelligence organizing it. How we organize our thoughts and emotions and what we do with them reflect our intelligence.

One of the main purposes of emotion in the human system is to provide a means of expression for core heart feelings. But since heart intelligence isn't developed in most people, the mind more often hijacks our emotional energy and uses it to express its perceptions and reactions.

When we let our unmanaged thoughts dictate how we respond emotionally, we're asking for trouble. In addition, emotional memories and reactions can operate at a subconscious level and influence our thought processes. Our subconscious emotional system can trigger a feeling faster than the mind can intercept it. [5] That's why we often experience feelings without knowing why. And even when we *do* know why, and try to manage our emotional reaction, we can't; emotions are simply too fast. The rational mind by itself doesn't have the ability to intervene in ways that produce helpful results. The disorder of an unmanaged mind combined with the power of unmanaged emotion often creates an internal war. We get caught in a depleting internal argument that can go on for hours.

*Example 1:* Jeff is in a restaurant when an elderly man walks by and knocks over his coffee, splashing the hot liquid all over his suit and tie. Rationally, he knows that the man couldn't help himself, so Jeff says, "That's okay, don't worry about it." But in his feeling world, he's having a fit. His thoughts are screaming, "Look at my suit! What am I going to do? How can I go back to the office with coffee stains all over my clothes?" Jeff is reacting at two different levels—reason and emotion. Each level has its own perspective, and if Jeff lets them, they'll fight each other all afternoon.

In this case it would be energy-efficient for Jeff to stop pretending that everything is okay and recognize that his emotions aren't in balance. He could then do a quick FREEZE-FRAME to rebalance his nervous system and heart rhythms, activating a core heart feeling such as appreciation or compassion to stop the energy drain before it colors the rest of his day. From a point of heart coherence, he would then have the power to take some of the significance and emotional energy out of the issue, reassuring himself that things like this happen to everyone at one time or another. When he asked himself, "What would be a more efficient response to the situation, one that would minimize future stress?" his intuition, common sense, and sincerity would tell him that people back at the office aren't going to judge him for coffee stains on his clothes and that he'll easily be able to get his suit cleaned the next day. In this state of head/heart alignment he can let the issue go completely.

*Example 2:* There's an incident at the office between Barbara and Dan, who are both stressed out trying to meet a deadline. They snap at each other, and everyone notices. Later, in thoughts and words, they exchange apologies. But in their respective feeling worlds, it may take all day for the dust to settle. Their rational minds are okay, but their feeling worlds aren't. It's the continued motion of energy in the feeling world, and the speed and momentum of that energy, that causes continued drain.

If the rational mind continues to say that everything's fine when it's not, the emotional drain goes on, placing a cloud over our quality of life and slowly damaging our health. After awhile we're left with a vague awareness of feeling bad but no accompanying thoughts that would explain why.

If Barbara and Dan would stop to connect with their heart intelligence, they could reduce the time it'll take to regain emotional balance. Sooner or later they'll forget about the incident anyway, of course, but they'll lose a lot of energy along the way if they ignore the need to come back into alignment in the moment. By making the effort to engage with the heart, and even trying to activate a core heart feeling of nonjudgment or forgiveness, they could access the power and self-awareness needed to release the unresolved emotions around their tense exchange and stop the energy drain. It takes effort to shift to the heart and gain the coherence to let go of inefficient thoughts and emotions, but as heart intelligence is developed, that process gets easier.

## The Cascade Effect

Each person's entire emotional history is logged into his or her neural circuitry and imprinted in memory. Thus an emotional response in the present can trigger a cascade of associated emotional memories, adding more fuel to the fire. If we were hurt in the past by someone we loved, we can become paranoid about getting hurt by others who show us love. Sometimes even the smallest reaction can cause a download of associated emotions from prior incidents. Old grudges, lingering bits of unforgiveness, unpleasant associations, and unresolved fears can become amplified by the most trivial issues.

Because of this cascade effect, we're usually dealing not just with the emotions of the moment but also with the accumulation of emotional experiences stored in our emotional memory banks. And there are physiological reasons for this.

Deep inside the brain is a processing center called the amygdala, which is responsible for assigning emotional significance to everything we hear, smell, touch, and see. [6] The amygdala can influence and be influenced by information from our cerebral cortex, and it's also influenced by input from the heart. [7]

Neuroscientist Dr. Karl Pribram explains in his book *Brain and Perception* how the amygdala compares what's *familiar* in memory with new information coming into the brain. [8] If an old emotion has become familiar, we often respond to new, similar situations with the same emotion, whether it makes sense or not. In a strange way, the familiarity makes us feel secure.

For example, a boy who lives in a house where there's frequent yelling and violence develops emotions of insecurity and a pervading sense of fear. At school, if a classmate raises his voice or even looks questioningly at the boy, that action can trigger the familiar sense of fear. Perceiving the current situation from a perspective of familiarized fear, he may react with more aggression than is warranted, perhaps even hitting the classmate. Emotionally, his response would feel like self-defense; he's doing what he deems appropriate to feel secure. For the same reason, when this boy grows up he may resort to violence and abuse with his own family.

The amygdala eavesdrops on incoming information flowing through our brains, searching for anything that has emotional significance. All of us have had the experience of meeting someone and disliking him immediately without apparent cause. Maybe he evokes the unconscious memory of a schoolteacher who always picked on us in class, even though we can't remember the guy's name. The amygdala assigns significance very rapidly, but not always very accurately.

For decades it was thought that all information from the senses went first to the cerebral cortex, where it was mentally analyzed, and then to the amygdala for emotional assessment. Only recently have neuroscientists discovered a brain circuit that lets our perceptions go directly through to the amygdala *without* passing through the rational decision-making area of the cortex. [5] That's why the boy from the abusive household may feel his heart pounding and adrenaline surging whenever someone raises his voice, though he may not even realize that the raised voice reminds him of his father.

## Where Do Emotions Come From?

W hen parts of the brain are damaged or surgically removed in older children and adults, those people can no longer experience certain emotions. For that reason, many scientists have concluded that emotions originate only in the brain.

Another group of scientists believe that emotions are created only through biochemistry. This would imply that we're completely at the mercy of our biochemical experience, however—that we have no choice regarding our emotional experience. And it doesn't explain why electrical and biochemical changes in the brain very often occur in response to emotions and perceptions over which we *do* have choice.

The latest evidence shows that it works *both* ways. Candace Pert, M.D., author of *Molecules of Emotions*, concludes that our biochemistry affects our emotional responses, but our emotions affect our biochemistry in return. Dr. Pert reveals that biochemicals are actually the physiological correlates of emotions. The molecules of emotion run every system in our body via a communication system that clearly demonstrates a body/mind intelligence. [9]

Our brain circuits are shaped by our experiences throughout life. Thus it's never too late for change and growth. We've found that the heart is the most powerful agent for emotional change in the body. Here's why.

Information from our heart finds its way to the amygdala. In fact, the cells in the amygdala exhibit electrical activity that's synchronized to the heartbeat. As the heartbeat changes, so does the electrical activity in the cells of the amygdala. [10] This may explain why positive changes in feeling and perception occur when heart rhythms become more coherent as people use the HeartMath Solution tools and techniques. [10–14]

A recent cardiological study showed that 55 percent of participants who experienced symptoms of panic disorder actually had an undiagnosed heart arrhythmia that triggered the feelings of panic. In the majority of these cases, once the heart arrhythmia was treated, the panic disorder went away. If their arrhythmias hadn't been discovered, all of these people would have been sent to a psychiatrist for treatment. [15]

## Overcoming Emotional History

Ordinarily, when we set out to eliminate emotional baggage, we look to various psychotherapeutic techniques. Among the most common choices are psychoanalysis, behavioral modification, and cognitive therapy. Our new understandings of the function of the brain and heart give us clues as to how these approaches work.

According to Joseph LeDoux, a leading authority in neuroscience, it's believed that these three major therapies each help the cortex override the amygdala, but they use different neural pathways to do it. [5]

Behavioral and cognitive therapies teach patients new behaviors, primarily depending on the interaction between the prefrontal cortex and the amygdala. Psychoanalysis, on the other hand, requires patients to achieve conscious insight into their behavior. To do that, it delves into memories stored in the temporal lobe and the cortical areas related to consciousness.

Because it seeks to eliminate emotional baggage and other more serious disorders by achieving conscious insight into memories, psychoanalysis is inherently a longer process. And it's not an easy one: as we've said, emotional memories can distort perceptions and override conscious thoughts. This is in part because within the wiring of the brain, the neural connections from the emotional system to the cognitive system are stronger and more numerous than the connections going from the cognitive to the emotional system. [5] At every step of the way, then, conscious thinking can be overcome by powerful, amygdala-driven emotion.

Because our emotional history and reactions can be triggered unconsciously and then bypass the mind's reasoning process, it takes a power stronger than the mind to change emotional patterning. Our theory is that when conscious insight does occur, in any type of therapeutic process, it's because the coherent power and intelligence of the heart have become engaged.

The most effective therapists know that it's through a heart connection that patients experience their deepest "aha" moments and insights. That heart connection can be initiated through the caring and sensitive communication of a therapist, or it can come about as the patient connects with her own core heart feelings.

On the basis of the Institute's research, we're suggesting that a more direct route to emotional freedom can be achieved by helping patients consciously go to the heart first. In going directly to the heart by using FREEZE-FRAME, applying CUT-THRU, or activating a core heart feeling, people often have intuitive perception shifts that help them find release. They don't necessarily have to bring up or relive old emotional memories. Rehashing emotional memories more often than not *reinforces* those memories in the cells of the brain. Thus that process, instead of bringing us the insights we need to release old memories from our system, often reignites the mind's justification and hurt, creating more incoherence. When we're trying to work through a long-standing, emotionally charged issue, reinforcing memories isn't a means of resolution. We need to access the heart's deeper intelligence.

As knowledge of heart intelligence increases in the therapeutic community, doctors and patients alike will benefit by learning to access their hearts in the first place and then proceed from there. By engaging heart intelligence, therapists will have greater intuitive insight on how to guide their patients, and patients will have greater power and intuitive insight on how to release emotional history and keep the past from conditioning perceptions and reactions.

A benchmark of emotional management and responsibility is the realization that our past can no longer be blamed for our actions in the present. While it's important to acknowledge emotional history, we shouldn't give in to the tendency to use our past to excuse our current behavior. Despite good intentions, a lot of people committed to personal growth *know* that they shouldn't do that, but they lack the power to stop themselves. They wander off down a sidetrack, feeling sorry for themselves and blaming other people.

With the pace of change and stress accelerating, people won't have time for sidetracks much longer. They're too costly in time and energy. The ability to quickly shift out of negative emotional states, past or present, into new understanding and insight is on the horizon. Though it represents a quantum leap from working things out incrementally, it's not as far off in the future as we may think.

As you practice the HeartMath Solution tools and concepts, you'll gain the power and intelligence you need. The tools will help you become more aware of your thoughts, emotions, attitudes, actions, and reactions. As you practice them, you'll develop a keen assessment of mental and emotional assets and deficits. You'll see where you allow yourself to mechanically adopt attitudes or hold on to mind-sets that entrap you in emotional discord. By engaging the power of your heart each step of the way, the tools will help you build emotional coherence and achieve more control over the direction of your life.

## A New Level of Mastery

At HeartMath, we foresee that the next major step in the evolution of the human species will necessitate the development of a higher degree of emotional management than we've ever experienced. This level of emotional management, this application of heart intelligence, will be the root of our power for profound personal and societal change.

We've all experienced managing our emotions to some degree. But what we usually practice is a kind of "fair-weather management." When the sun is shining and the sky is clear, we can smile and feel emotionally balanced. But when a storm appears—especially one that wasn't forecast—our emotions are thrown into turmoil. We're basically at the mercy of our inner environment.

When life conforms to the standards set by our minds, it's easy to keep a light rein on our emotions and still feel pretty good. But if one little thing happens that we think *shouldn't* have happened, it's over. We haven't yet learned the skills to move to the next level emotionally. We're still like adolescents.

If you gave a bunch of eager ten-year olds the keys to your car, they'd be happy to drive it, but they wouldn't know how. When they got behind the wheel and drove off, there's a good chance they'd have a wreck. That's where many of us are when it comes to managing emotions. We don't know how to manage how we feel, so year after year we suffer the consequences.

Most of us are doing the best we can. But emotional management has to be carefully cultivated, and unfortunately there aren't many instruction manuals. For the most part, people learn through a trial-and-error process—the school of hard knocks. They master enough emotional management skills to survive and to conform to social norms, but they can't consciously orchestrate emotions well enough to "drive" effectively.

Let's look at a simple example of how unmanaged emotions can drive us into the ditch. You wake up on a Saturday and decide to take a peaceful drive in the country. It's an impulsive decision, and since you usually plan things carefully, you feel pleased with yourself—so pleased that you forget to gas up the car. Five miles down an absolutely gorgeous mountain road in the middle of nowhere, you run out of gas.

"How could this *happen?*" you groan. "Things were going so well!"

You look for someone to blame—and you're the only one around: "I can't believe I was so stupid!" On your five-mile walk back to civilization, blame gives way to self-pity: "Every time I try to do something fun and spontaneous there's a problem." Then fear and anxiety take over: "I remember passing some buildings five miles back, but was there a gas station?" Finally panic and despair set in: "What if this turns out to be a *twenty*-mile walk? What if someone vandalizes my car while I'm gone?"

Here's a better what-if: What if, at any point along the road, you'd been able to engage your heart intelligence, giving you more emotional control and a balanced reaction to the situation—one that didn't take you into blame, self-pity, fear, and panic? What if you'd remembered to FREEZE-FRAME as soon as you started to feel your emotions begin to boil? Not only would you have saved a lot of energy, but you would've been developing emotional management skills that could come in handy a hundred times a day.

Instead of feeling disappointment, self-judgment, and anxiety about the incident, with a one-minute FREEZE-FRAME you could have shifted from a stressful response into a state of neutral; perhaps you could even have see your predicament as fun, relaxing, and regenerative. The walk to the gas station on a beautiful day in the mountains might have been quite enjoyable, under other circumstances. Without emotional stress coloring the perception of the event, you might easily have seen the gift in it all. Remember, stress is a matter of *perception*.

Life is filled with mistakes, accidents, people who don't do what we want, and things we can't control. But we *can* control our emotions. Having control over our emotions in a positive, healthy way can make all the difference.

Emotional intelligence implies the ability to self-regulate our moods, control our impulses, delay gratification, persist despite frustration, and motivate ourselves. It includes empathy for others and the buoyancy of hope. [16] When we're equipped with those strengths, the twists and turns of life don't get us down. We roll with them.

We tend to think that further development of the head and reason will help us manage our emotions, but reason is what got us into emotional despair on that five-mile journey to find a gas station. It takes the heart-directed head to provide commonsense reasoning.

Heart intelligence helps us realize that we don't have to blame ourselves, the weather, or anyone else for our emotional experiences; we can adjust and regulate our emotions ourselves. The coherent power of the heart helps us perceive what to do and gives us poise and balance. Remember, heart intelligence isn't something sentimental or overly sweet. It has a businesslike quality; it's balanced, it's efficient, and it takes all possibilities into consideration. From a perspective of well-developed heart intelligence, it's easy to see that not expressing anger at someone doesn't mean that we accept or condone her behavior. And not judging ourselves—not feeling guilty or wallowing in self-pity—doesn't mean that we don't want to grow from our mistakes. If we listen to the heart and follow its directives, we can make the choice to manage our emotions early on in the reactive process, without getting sucked into a downward spiral.

## Positive Thinking Versus Positive *Feeling*

As a young man, I (Doc) used to love reading Norman Vincent Peale's books on the power of positive thinking. Although I enjoyed practicing Peale's positive affirmations, sometimes my emotional world got in a funk and refused to go along with my positive thoughts. I could change my thoughts but not my mood.

As I embarked on my research into the human heart, I realized that people are more a product of their feeling world than their thinking world. I concluded that the biblical saying, "As a [person] thinketh in his heart, so is he," would have had a very different meaning if it said, "As a person thinketh in his *head*."

Imagine a group of people who practice positive thinking driving to the country for a picnic. They enjoy each other's company and have a pleasant drive, but they can't help but notice the clouds forming overhead.

By the time they get to the picnic area, it's raining. "So," they tell each other, "here's a chance to practice our positive thinking. Let's not worry about it. We can have a picnic another time." That's a nice, positive thought. But their feelings are saying something quite different. These folks have just taken a long, pointless drive in the rain, and they feel disappointment and regret in equally large measure. Those feelings aren't bad or wrong. They reflect human nature. But there's another solution.

By pausing to go to their hearts, and using a HeartMath tool to activate the power of core heart feelings, they could shift their feeling state and tap into the wisdom of their hearts. Activating core heart feelings would introduce a much deeper emotional experience—perhaps gratitude for each other, the fun of being together, and the joy of unexpected moments. Surrounded by emotions like that, it's easier to see that disappointment and regret are not worth the energy. Instead of having to try to affirm themselves or grudgingly talk themselves out of thinking and feeling a certain way, by shifting perception to a wider picture they can release disappointment and regret quite naturally.

The power to change or transcend our feeling world comes from within us, from our own heart relaying its intelligence through our emotions. It's not about trying to affirm or reason our way into emotional intelligence. Without heart alignment, we'd chase that dream forever. Heart intuition or intelligence brings the freedom and power to accomplish what the mind—even with all the disciplines and affirmations in the world—can't do if it's out of sync with the heart.

## Preset Patterns

When something throws you off, you can *react* from the head or *act* from the heart. It's not always easy to stop the head, but activating heart power enables you to delay reacting and slide into neutral more freely, without letting subtle emotions get the best of you.

Life is full of opportunities that encourage us to give up trying to become more emotionally balanced. Society is entrained as a whole to the mismanagement of emotions. In this environment, it can be especially challenging to do something original, to act effectively rather than react predictably.

We call our individual or social reaction patterns "presets." Someone does us wrong, and predictably we fall into habit patterns ingrained in our emotional psyche and reinforced by societal programming. Someone pushes our buttons, and all those well-worn neural circuits kick in, triggering a preset reaction before we even know what hit us. That's where almost everybody gets stuck.

Presets are entrenched responses such as, "My father *always* makes me angry when he says that!" or "I'll *never* forget what my ex-wife did!" After months or years of practice, these patterns have so much force and stability that we need as much energy to overcome them as we invested in the first place—if not more. That's why we need an accumulation of heart power to change them.

### The Major Energy-Draining Presets

Two major presets can quickly compromise our efforts at emotional management: justification and principle.

Both of these mind-sets can seem so right. We feel good about it when we're "justifiably" angry, hurt, hostile, disappointed, or intolerant. Then, after we're drained by those emotions, we blame the person or situation we were "justifiably" upset about for making us feel bad. But we've already seen, in Chapter 3, that our bodies don't make a distinction between the times we're in the right and the times we're in the wrong. Even if we could prove to the whole world that we were right, our bodies still wouldn't care. Our heart rhythms and our nervous, hormonal, and immune systems would respond the same way they would if we knew we were wrong. Justified or not, emotions that cause stress — those that are sometimes labeled "negative" — simply aren't healthy. They deplete our emotional bank account, making it harder for us to regain emotional balance, and they inhibit our reasoning abilities.

Because the cascade effect of emotions throughout the body doesn't depend on whether emotions are justified or not, we prefer to call emotions that add coherence and energy to our system "asset emotions" and emotions that cause incoherence and deplete energy "deficit emotions," rather than labeling them "positive" or "negative" — terms that imply right or wrong, good or bad. The biological reality is more neutral than that. From the body's point of view, emotions aren't right or wrong, but we can say that they're either efficient or inefficient for our health and quality of life.

### The Justification Trap

Indulging in justification is an obvious, natural mistake. In fact, justification is the number-one reason that people don't successfully manage emotions.

Like fair-weather management, justification implies that we need to manage our emotions only under certain circumstances — not, for instance, when it's "understandable" that we got mad or frustrated. If we have a good reason to feel hurt, then we don't need to manage our tears of disappointment or blame and we don't need to try to work the issue out with the other person. Understandable or not, justification simply costs us too much.

When we suspend our emotional management because we have reasons that "excuse" our emotional indulgences, the aftereffect is like pollution or secondhand smoke in our system. It creates cross-currents in our feeling world that we then have to spend valuable time and energy clearing out.

As we become more observant of what goes on internally, we can see the progression: justified reaction, emotional drain, backwash of more depleting thoughts and emotions about the same issue, overload, more drain, then blame.

For some people, this emotional progression starts before they get out of the shower in the morning. One justified reaction to mere *thoughts* in the shower — about how much we have to do, how the day is going to go, or what someone did yesterday that we didn't like — and the emotional backwash starts. Then we spend the next few hours trying to feel better and recoup our lost energy — and wondering what truck hit us.

It's easy to become trapped in this process unless we realize how deficit emotions work. With that understanding, though, we can start to notice that one or two of these progressions in a day leaves us significantly less energy to appreciate and enjoy what we value in life.

### The Principle of the Thing

Let's look at the second major preset that compromises emotional management. Very often our justified reactions are based on our mind's adherence to principles. We justify our rude response to someone because "he shouldn't have talked to me that way." We justify the debris on the kitchen floor by telling ourselves, and anyone else who will listen, "It's not that I can't take out the trash. It's that *she* should take it out once in awhile. It's just the principle of the thing."

Sticking to principles can ensnare us in a morass of deficit emotions. If we hide behind self-righteousness, we separate ourselves from our heart and our potential connection to others.

There's nothing wrong with having high standards. Principles build character and integrity and provide a useful baseline for guiding our decisions and behavior. But if our sense of principle is used to sanction being judgmental, resentful, or indignant because something isn't right or fair in our eyes, then "principle" isn't working for us. It's going to deplete us quickly.

Sometimes we think of "righteous anger"—anger in defense of principle—as good anger. But it creates the same incoherence as any other anger. Unless it's taken to the heart and transformed into coherence, it blocks effective solutions.

Sometimes we think that we can't take needed action, whether in a confrontation or in getting something important done, without being propelled by anger. While anger can give us a short burst of energy, until we manage the anger we can't see what action would be best to take. The information is simply not available to us. The emotions have short-circuited the pathway in the brain that helps us see the most appropriate action.

We all know people who say, "It's the principle of the matter," to justify the toxic emotions they've sustained for years. As they hold onto their anger or hurt, they bleed away their energy reserves, often ending up bitter and depressed.

We knew an eighty-year-old man, the eldest of eleven siblings, who died lonely and bitter because he refused to make amends with his one remaining living brother. Forty years earlier, he'd stopped talking to this brother because he hadn't asked him to be part of a business investment that included another brother. The old man had never met this offending brother's grandchildren, and he'd avoided parties and family gatherings where he'd be present. It was the *principle* of the matter. How many destructive family feuds and years of misery are based on principle?

## Dealing with Energy-Draining Presets

*Any* rationalization of deficit emotions—whether it's based on justification or principle—traps our emotional energy in hurt, blame, fear, disappointment, betrayal, regret, remorse, or guilt. These attitudes tend to last a long time, because we continually rejustify them. Thus their devastation is cumulative.

What we may not anticipate is that, as they slowly drain our energy reserves, they leave us more vulnerable to *new* emotional drains. Yet rationalizing our emotions with justification or principle often starts with just a few seemingly innocent thoughts that we let ourselves get worked up over. For instance, how often do we find ourselves thinking or making statements such as these:

"I'm not mad; I'm just hurt."

"I'm not upset; I'm just disappointed."

"It's just not fair."

"I've been misunderstood."

"It's the principle of the thing."

"I have a right to be hurt [or angry or to feel betrayed]."

"If only I'd just . . . "

Though this type of inner dialogue seems normal, it's like a car tachometer that's missing its red warning line. If left unchecked, it can lead to serious consequences. In fact, much of the emotional stress in the world is ignited by this type of inner dialogue.

When people and situations don't satisfy our mental expectations, it's easy to rationalize our emotional behavior. And the statement, "I'm not upset; I'm just disappointed," implies a certain degree of emotional management. But even disappointment means resignation to emotional drain. You've merely traded a stronger emotion—being upset—for a lesser one. Being upset costs you more energy than being disappointed, so you come out a little ahead in the short term—but not by much, and not in the long run.

It's tricky, because the mind can justify being disappointed longer than it can justify being angry and upset. The stronger deficit emotions throw our mental, nervous, hormonal, and immune systems out of balance to the point that it's obvious we need to do something. The body compensates, fighting to bring itself back to normal, when stressed by strong deficit emotions. Getting upset burns a lot of energy physically, mentally, and especially emotionally. Eventually we simply run out of the emotional energy needed to sustain the upset.

Disappointment, on the other hand, is less intense. Although disappointment has a depleting effect on our physiology, it's more subtle and takes less energy to sustain. So we let disappointment linger, often until it bleeds into sadness. And then sustained sadness bleeds into depression or despair. Because the initial feeling is justified, you may not notice that disappointment is setting you up to experience more disappointments and draining emotions.

Hurt works the same way. The very term "hurt feelings" implies an inward drain of emotional energy. Like disappointment, hurt can also linger and progress into blame, anger, grief, guilt, and other draining attitudes. It's time to stop the drain, time for us to understand how emotions work and realize that we have new choices in how we respond to them.

So what do we do? Innocent people do get hurt. People do misunderstand us and disappoint us. Freeing ourselves from justified feelings of betrayal requires a courageous act of self-care. It takes new awareness and the power of the heart to release, let go, and move on. An understanding of how thoughts and emotions work is what gives us the new intelligence and motivation we need.

First of all, if you recognize yourself in the inner dialogue statements given above, don't worry or get stressed about it. We all make these statements sometimes. Just realize that they represent common, stress-producing attitudes that remain hidden behind a cloak of justification. Once you remove the cloak, you can begin to identify patterns that ignite your emotional stress, and then you can use your heart intelligence to change them.

## A Laundromat Story

Years ago, when I (Doc) was sitting in a laundromat in North Carolina waiting for my clothes to dry, I saw two women I knew, Maude and Cassie, standing over by the dryers, fanning themselves and gossiping.

I heard one of them explaining that she'd lent Billy and Margo, a couple she knew from church, three thousand dollars to help pay for some unexpected medical bills.

"They said they'd pay me back in three months," Maude said, sighing. "But it's been five months now, Cassie, and they haven't given me any money. It looks like they're avoiding me."

Cassie looked uncomfortable for a minute, trying to make up her mind, and then said, "Maude, I heard that they did pay some money to the hospital. But I also heard that they used the rest to build that new deck onto their house. Billy hasn't been working much lately. They just don't have the money to pay you back right now."

I watched as Maude tried her best to manage her emotions. She gathered herself up not to react.

"Well, I'm just not going to get worked up about it," she said firmly, speaking mostly to herself. "They know where to find me when they get back on their feet. It's better just to let it go and hope for the best."

"That's good," Cassie said. "There's nothing you can do about it right now anyway."

Neither one of them spoke for several minutes. Then suddenly Maude blurted out, "I'm not *mad* at them. But I don't understand how they could build a new deck with that money. It kind of hurts my feelings. Just when you trust somebody. It's . . . disappointing."

Maude knew she didn't want to get upset about the situation, but putting a cork on her emotions didn't seem to be working. They spilled over anyway. Her first response had been anger. When that made her uncomfortable, she tried to stave it off by insisting that she wasn't mad.

I watched Cassie to see what she'd say next, what advice she might give, but she kept her eyes cast down and folded her clothes deliberately. The sound of the washers and dryers roared over their uncomfortable silence.

Still grappling with her emotions, Maude tried to turn things on herself. "I guess I should have seen it coming. How could I be so stupid? I've got nobody to blame but myself."

Trying to deal with feeling taken advantage of, she soon lashed out at her friend: "Cassie, if you knew about this, why didn't you tell me sooner? Why didn't you stop me from giving them money if you knew they were like that?"

Cassie mumbled something inaudible as they packed up their clothes and walked out of the laundromat. The last thing I heard was Maude saying sternly, "Well, I'm not going to put up with this. It's just not right, and I've got every reason in the world to be mad as hell about it."

Watching this woman suffer as she fought to control her emotions made me feel deep compassion for her. She went through an emotional progression I'd seen so often: first hurt, then anger, then disappointment, then guilt or resentment, then betrayal, and finally justified fury. Though the anger rankled, she'd probably been taught from childhood that getting mad was wrong. Besides, she had a sweet temperament—I could see that she didn't like feeling angry—and she could probably see how uncomfortable the anger made her friend. So she was up against personal and social imperatives to feel something else. And she made a valiant effort to fend the anger off before giving in.

If Maude had had tools to tap into her heart intelligence, she could have eliminated her struggle altogether. Anyone hearing that her trust had been betrayed would have been alarmed. Anger is a natural response to news like that. But knowing that anger prevents us from thinking clearly, intuitively, and objectively, and knowing its destructive impact on the body, we don't have to either indulge it or repress it. We can do something different.

Stepping back from Cassie's news and consulting her heart intelligence, Maude might have realized that (1) Cassie might not have had her facts right, and (2) even if Cassie was accurate, the betrayal probably wasn't a personal insult. Billy and Margo were probably just being irresponsible again. Maybe they *did* take advantage of her, but they still intended to pay her back. If Maude had asked her heart for advice about how to handle this betrayal, she might have come up with some very firm guidelines to present to Billy and Margo.

At the very least, heart intelligence gives us the power to delay emotional reactivity until we have all the facts. Emotional management doesn't mean that we acquiesce to whatever happens to us. On the contrary, we often have to stand up for ourselves and take action. But heart intelligence helps us see what to do cleanly and clearly, with less suffering.

Progress can be made in releasing emotional issues if we identify each issue and take back the power we've invested in it. Our heart can show us a healthier response to any of these unmanaged emotions. It comes fully equipped with the ability to give us the awareness to make new choices and move on. The high-speed, intuitive intelligence of the heart can quickly help us see where we're compromising our emotional integrity and give us the power to do something about it.

## Taking the Significance Out

If you asked a hundred adults to spend a day with four- and five-year-olds at a day-care center, it wouldn't be long before they started using heart intelligence without even thinking about it.

In a large group of kids that age, it's never long before one starts to cry. Perhaps his toy is broken. Or perhaps other kids have taken the wagon and left him behind. Either situation seems like the end of the world. Most adults would try to calm the child by helping him put things in perspective. The toy can be fixed, they say. The other kids will be back soon. For adults, it's instinctual to help children take the significance out of problems.

The same thing happens with teenagers. Say you're visiting a family with a couple of teenagers who are upset because their parents won't let them go to a concert. One is angry and acting out; the other is crying. Hoping that you can persuade their parents to let them go, the kids turn to you for support. The first thing you try to do to calm them is help them reduce the significance. You show them different ways to look at the situation and different approaches to take with their parents. On your way home, you may tell yourself that someone needs to show those kids how to manage their emotions. Your common sense tells you that when too much significance is assigned to any situation, there's an enormous emotional energy waste.

Taking the significance out of issues and events is second nature to adults dealing with children. But we don't tend to offer that same help to ourselves. Instead, we do what most kids do—argue, pout, and blame. But if taking the significance out works for kids, it'll work for us too. And when we do turn that tool on ourselves, the results are powerful.

Emotions have to be checked in the moment or they cascade. It's the *extra* significance and the *ongoing* emotional investment that we put into an issue that make us feel we're going to blow up. Our reactions are no different than a child's tantrum. Sometimes we intuitively know that we need to let go of a deficit emotion but can't make the shift because of what we might call a "mind pout." We cut off our nose to spite our face: we know that we're depleting our system, but we just won't release the significance. We develop an *attachment* to the drain and give way to a mind pout.

The trouble is that when we ignore one deficit emotion and refuse to take the significance out even after we're aware of it, the emotional depletion builds, undermining our progress in other areas. The next thing we know, we feel a sense of guilt and failure. *Nothing*'s working. It seems hard to make any progress; we feel as if we're taking two steps forward, three steps back. Soon we're feeling sorry for ourselves.

In reality, it was just that one initial thing that went wrong, starting the drain, but now it feels as if *everything*'s gone wrong. If we go back and isolate the precipitating thing and take the significance out of that, we replenish our energy and free ourselves to notice and appreciate the other things we've made progress on.

Many people cave in to emotional drains, offering the popular excuse that "they just can't help it." It's time now that we learn both how and why to "help it"—or at least become open to the fact that we *can*. Emotional management means knowing when to cut loss and take action to self-restore our system by mustering our own heart intelligence to do something different. To take the significance out, we have to call on our own higher self: the wisdom coming through the heart.

## Approach It with Heart

The tools of the HeartMath Solution will help you reroute your feelings through the heart so that the energy drains that are invisibly depleting your system stop. Each time you use a tool, you build your heart's capacity to get back into an intuitive flow. Emotions liquefied become flow, and mind aligned with heart becomes intuition.

As you develop the connection with your heart, that organ of intelligence will assure you that refined emotional behavior is within your grasp. You'll learn to ease uncomfortable emotions out through the heart and increase coherence so that the intuition of your heart becomes louder and clearer. Soon you'll be identifying and acknowledging emotions and taking the significance out of problems naturally.

Managing emotions and getting them in balance has to be approached in steps. If you have a tendency to be angry, acknowledge the anger, then balance it by easing back to the heart and using FREEZE-FRAME. This creates a window of opportunity for intuition to come in from the heart and do what the mind can't do—whether because of discipline or repression. Intuition is freeing and can present you alternative perceptions and new responses to anger.

Understandably, there may be moments when you feel a little apprehensive. All of us quail at taking an unguarded look at our own emotions, afraid that we'll come across something that's hard to accept or control. Our emotions are in Pandora's box, and we want to keep the lid on.

At moments like that, it takes courage to take on our emotions, but the effort is worth it. Luckily, courage is associated with the heart. By using tools that tap into the power of the heart, we're positioned to draw on an inner courage that we may not even have known we had.

Here are some tips that can help you improve your emotional management:

- Start using the HeartMath tools on small drains and go to the heart for resolution as those drains come up.

- Use FREEZE-FRAME with consistency and ask your heart to help you see where you're falling into fair-weather management or reacting based on justification or principle.

- Call on the heart's transformative power to take the significance out of issues so that you don't let emotional deficits stack up.

- If you have a setback, don't be hard on yourself. Take the significance out, go right back to the heart, and start again. Give your heart intelligence a chance to offer its perspectives and solutions. That's treating yourself with emotional balance and maturity.

- Try not to think of emotional management as something to dread — just one more thing you have to do. It's exciting to know that you can move quickly to your next level of fulfillment by applying heart to your emotions.

When emotions are managed by the heart, they heighten your awareness of the world around you and add sparkle to life. The result is new intelligence and a new view of life. Just be sincere in your efforts and appreciate the progress you make, not expecting to be free from unpleasant emotions all at once. Each success builds more power and excitement. It gets easier as you go. When long-standing emotional issues lose some of their intensity and importance, things won't bother you as much.

With just a little effort to unlock your heart intelligence, you'll begin to experience an exciting new freedom. Your emotional experiences will become substantially more pleasurable, and you'll begin to feel textures in the heart that you've never felt before. People everywhere who are trying to follow their hearts are confirming this. They're comparing notes and discovering similar exciting results. And as you progress, experiencing more and more of those rewarding textures, the progress itself will become a powerful motivation to keep unraveling the mysteries of emotion.

## KEY POINTS TO REMEMBER

➤ The emotional frontier is truly the next frontier to conquer in human understanding. The opportunity we face now, even before that frontier is fully explored and settled, is to develop our emotional potential and accelerate rather dramatically into a new state of being.

➢ Emotional energy works at a higher speed than the speed of thought. This is because your feeling world operates at a higher speed than your mind.

➢ Emotions in themselves aren't really intelligent. But anything that has a flow—as emotion and thought do—has an organizing intelligence behind it.

➢ People approach life from the perspective of familiarized emotional reactions stored in the amygdala of the brain, and they respond with familiarized behavior in an attempt to feel secure.

➢ A benchmark of new emotional management lies in realizing that our past can no longer be blamed for our actions in the present.

➢ There are two major mind-sets that quickly compromise efforts at emotional management: justification and principle. These mind-sets trap your emotional energy in hurt, blame, fear, disappointment, betrayal, regret, remorse, and/or guilt, which create cumulative drain and deficits in your system.

➢ One of the main keys to emotional management is learning to quickly arrest a draining or deficit emotion and generate an attitude shift from a place of deep heart maturity.

➢ To reclaim the energy out of a deficit emotion, we have to take out the significance we've assigned to it (or that our amygdala has assigned to it). To take the significance out, we first make an effort to back off; then the heart can open up.

➢ HeartMath Solution tools help you reroute your feeling-world memories, purifying them through the heart so the drains stop. Each time you use a tool, you build heart capacity to get back to an intuitive flow. Emotions liquefied become flow, and mind aligned with heart becomes intuition.

➢ As heart-based emotions and textures begin to replace old patterns, you'll feel a whole lot better. Experiencing more and more of those rewarding textures becomes a powerful motivation to keep unraveling the mystery of emotion.

# CHAPTER 8

# Care Versus Overcare

One day in fourth grade, I (Howard) was happily entertaining myself with spit wads at the back of the classroom. Like many a child before me, I somehow believed that the teacher wouldn't notice. But before too long she'd had enough. She took me to the old stucco wall at the back of the room. (I think the wall was originally white, but by the time my class came along, it was three shades of brown.) The teacher handed me a small pail of water and a rag and told me to clean the dirt-encrusted wall.

As an energetic fourth-grader looking for an outlet, I tackled the problem with both hands. An hour later I was *still* working diligently, all my attention focused on getting the dirt out of the crevices in that rough stucco.

"You know," my teacher said casually, "if you work as hard at everything in life as you're working on that wall, you'll be a very successful man."

She wasn't trying to boost my morale with exaggerated praise or sugar-coating; she was making a simple, sincere statement of what she saw as fact. It was an act of genuine care, and I've remembered it my whole life.

We've all had experiences like that, where one heartfelt remark made all the difference. Sometimes such remarks come from people we respect and love, but not always. A considerate stranger may say something in passing that we think about for years. It's not the words or the person who says them that makes such experiences memorable; we remember them because of the care.

We're all accustomed to feeling a heightened sense of care for our loved ones. That's one of the most rewarding things about our important relationships. But the idea of taking that generous, openhearted feeling into the street is something else entirely. Caring just for the sake of caring—that can be scary.

In the mean, cruel world, we have to keep our guard up, right? We can't go around caring helter-skelter. A few nights of watching the news is enough to make anyone fearful and withdrawn. Before long, the paranoia shows up in slogans like "Look out for yourself!" and "Get them before they get you!"

Years ago, New York City was stereotyped as a place populated by residents who, even if the most hideous crime were being committed right in front of them, wouldn't try to stop it. Many Americans believed that New Yorkers, living in an aggressive environment with a high crime rate, had become jaded and self-protective; they were perceived as people who thought that caring would only get them into deeper trouble, who didn't want to "get involved."

Even though statistics have since proven that New Yorkers aren't as unwilling to lend a hand as they appeared to be from media reports, the loss of small, friendly communities has changed us all. We often don't bother to meet our neighbors or even know who they are. Instead of acting on our natural instinct to care, we keep our guard up. We tell ourselves that if we don't, people will take advantage of us. We worry that we'll "waste" our energy on someone who won't give us care in return. We believe that we can't *afford* to care. But in fact the opposite is true: we can't afford *not* to.

Care is a powerful motivator. It's one of the most important core heart feelings. Care inspires and gently reassures us. Lending us a feeling of security and support, it reinforces our connection with others. Not only is it one of the best things we can do for our health, but it *feels* good—whether we're giving or receiving it. Caring for someone or something has a regenerative, uplifting effect on us. The experience—a tangible one—goes directly to our hearts. And it's an experience that we can pass on to someone else.

When we care for someone, we often express our feelings quite naturally through touch. We automatically hug our friends or pat them on the back. In conversation, we might touch their arm to emphasize a point or share a joke. When we're introduced, even to a stranger, we shake the person's hand—a moment of contact that makes a connection.

Researchers at the Institute have discovered that connection is more profound than we'd thought. If we touch someone, the electrical energy from our heart is transmitted to the other person's brain, and vice versa. If we were to hook two people up to monitors while they connected, we'd be able to see the pattern of one person's cardiac electrical signal (as graphed on an ECG) show up in the other person's brain waves (as graphed on an EEG). [1, 2]

To see what we mean, look at Figure 8.1. See how the heart's signal in Person B is clearly reflected in the brain waves of Person A when the two research subjects are holding hands? Even when two subjects simply stand close together, without actually touching, we can detect a similar effect. [1, 2] These results have been confirmed by other laboratories. [3]

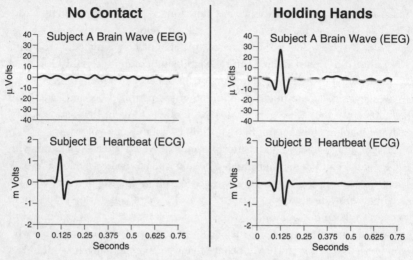

Heartbeat Signal Averaged Waveforms

*The Electricity of Touch*

FIGURE 8.1. Signal-averaging techniques were used to show that when two people touch, there's a transfer of the electrical energy generated by one person's heart (as represented by the tracings on an ECG) that can be detected in the other person's brain waves (via EEG).

© copyright 1998 Institute of HeartMath Research Center

These intriguing results show that when we touch someone else, an exchange of electromagnetic energy—from heart to brain—takes place. Whether we realize it or not, then, our hearts not only affect our own experience, but they can also influence those around us. In turn, we can be influenced by the signals that others send out. We shift to resonate with their energy, as they do with us. We aren't aware of this process, of course—at least not consciously. But it happens.

In Chapter 3 we learned that the frequency structure of the heart's electromagnetic field changes dramatically in different emotional states. Frustration produces an incoherent signal, while appreciation creates a harmonious, coherent one. Core heart feelings—care among them—generate coherence in the heart's field, while stressful feelings produce incoherence. [4] The resulting energy is transmitted throughout our bodies, and the fact that it radiates outside of the body as well has tremendous social implications.

Think about this. If those we touch or stand close to (say, in an elevator, a subway, or a department store) can pick up our heart's electromagnetic signal in their brain waves, we're in effect *broadcasting* our emotional states all the time (and receiving others').

Of course, we communicate emotional states in other ways as well; we learn to read each other through a complicated set of cues. Our mood is often apparent from our body language alone. But even without body language and additional cues, we transmit a subtle signal. We can't keep it in. All of us affect each other at the most basic electromagnetic level.

That means that the guy standing next to you in the checkout line may be more affected by how annoyed you are with your mother than either of you realize. And think of all the signals going back and forth in the crowds of people pushing their way into a rally or a rock concert. The implications are enormous.

We're only just beginning to understand the complicated connections between people. But it's already clear that if we touch someone while feeling an emotion like care, we're potentially transmitting a signal to that person's body that promotes well-being and health. [1]

Many doctors, nurses, and physical therapists are aware of the power of physical connection. There's growing scientific evidence of the benefits of caring touch. [5] Touch therapy, or massage, is as important to infants and children as eating and sleeping are, according to Dr. Tiffany Field, director of the Touch Research Institute at the University of Miami School of Medicine. [6]

Clinical studies have found that touch triggers physiological changes. Touch has been proved to help asthmatic children improve breathing function, diabetic children comply with treatment, and sleepless babies fall asleep with less trouble. [7] Caring touch is also helpful for adults' well-being and health. [8, 9] In some cases, the effect is decisive.

In a recent issue of the scientific journal *Subtle Energies*, Drs. Judith Green and Robert Shellenberger tell of an elderly woman who was dying of heart failure. When her physician realized that there was no more he could do for her, he called her family in for a last good-bye. Remarkably, the moment the family members touched her, her heartbeat resumed its normal rhythm. Half an hour later, she was alert and sitting up in bed. [10]

While not everyone recovers from a caring touch, the heart and brain still receive the signal. There may be other explanations for this elderly woman's recovery, and other contributing factors, but our studies on the electricity of touch have convinced us that the caring emotions of her family *could* have produced a discernible physiological effect—one powerful enough to encourage her heart.

## The Regenerative Power of Care

W ithout care, life loses its luster. When people "just don't care anymore," we can see the lack of vitality on their faces and in the way they walk and hold their bodies. We can even hear it in their voices. Without the regenerative energy of care running through their system, their bodies have no motive for maintaining themselves—literally, no reason to live.

On the other hand, care produces equally visible effects on the body—a bounce in the step, a gleam in the eye, and an inordinate enjoyment of the fleeting moments in life. Health and vitality spring from heart-based emotions such as care. And even if the evidence weren't so apparent, we could measure many of the physiological effects of care in the laboratory.

Even the experience of caring for an animal has been shown to improve morale and promote health in the elderly or those in nursing homes. Research supporting the health benefits of caring for pets ranges from the facilitation of social interaction to the physiological benefits of animals on cardiovascular responses. [11, 12]

Researchers at the Universities of Pennsylvania and Maryland found that a year after hospitalization for heart disease, the mortality rate of patients with pets was roughly one-third that of patients without pets. [13] Pets keep care an active part of millions of people's lives.

They also help youngsters learn how to care. Studies show that children with pets have a higher degree of empathy. [14] However, it's important to point out that the increased empathy is due not to the pet but to the sincere care that pets draw out. Pets are also a potential source of overcare and stress. It's how people respond to a pet that determines the regenerative benefit (or lack thereof).

## Vicarious and Self-Induced Care

I n the 1980s, David McClelland, a psychologist at Harvard, showed a group of subjects a video about Mother Teresa. As she moved among the poor and destitute, she was the embodiment of care and compassion.

To see if this vicarious experience would have an impact on his subjects, Dr. McClelland looked at their immune systems. We have an antibody called secretory IgA in our saliva and throughout our bodies. Our first line of defense against invading pathogens, it's an important measurement of immune system health. After the group watched the moving video, test results showed an immediate rise in secretory IgA levels. In other words, the feeling of care and compassion evoked in them by the video had a measurable effect on their immune systems. [15]

Interested in finding out whether "self-induced care" would have the same effect as vicarious care, Rollin McCraty and his team at the Institute of Heart-Math began by duplicating the McClelland study. They had very similar results. Immediately after watching the video, test subjects had an increase of 17 percent in IgA levels.

Then Rollin and his team took their research several steps further. They wanted to know whether feeling care without an external stimulus would have a greater or lesser effect. And what about other emotions? How would an experience of anger, for instance, compare to an experience of care? In addition, they were interested in finding out what the long-term effects of self-induced increases in IgA levels would be.

Test subjects were taught the FREEZE-FRAME technique and then asked to evoke a feeling of care and compassion for five minutes. Several days later, these same people were asked to feel five minutes of self-induced anger by remembering a situation or experience in their lives that had made them angry and recapturing the feeling as best they could. In both cases, IgA samples were taken immediately afterward and then every hour for six hours. Figure 8.2 illustrates the results.

After five minutes of feeling care and compassion, the subjects had an immediate 41 percent average increase in their IgA levels. After one hour, their IgA levels returned to normal, but then slowly *increased* over the next six hours. Rollin observed that self-induced care actually resulted in a larger rise in IgA than the vicarious feeling of care evoked by the Mother Teresa video. In some individuals, IgA increased as much as 240 percent immediately after they performed the FREEZE-FRAME technique.

There was also an immediate increase (18 percent) in IgA levels when the participants experienced anger. But an hour later, their IgA levels had dropped to only about half of what they were before the anger. Even after six hours, their IgA levels were still not back to normal. [16]

One five-minute experience of recalled anger and the effectiveness of our immune system is impaired for over *six hours*. Clearly, it takes a long time for our system to come back into balance once anger kicks in. And yet how many times each day are we faced with situations that have the potential to arouse

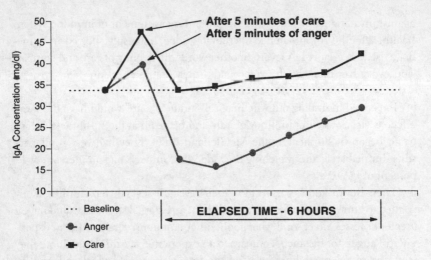

**The Impact of Anger Versus Care on the Immune System**

FIGURE 8.2. This graph compares the impact of one five-minute episode of recalled anger against that of a five-minute experience of care on the immune antibody secretory IgA over a six-hour period. When subjects recalled an angry feeling for five minutes, an initial slight increase in IgA was followed by a dramatic drop, which persisted for the following six hours (bottom trace). In contrast, when subjects used the FREEZE-FRAME technique and focused on feeling sincere care for five minutes, there was a significant increase in IgA, which returned to baseline an hour later and then slowly increased throughout the rest of the day (top trace).

© copyright 1998 Institute of HeartMath Research Center

anger? If simply *remembering* an angry feeling can have such an enormous impact on our defense mechanisms, imagine the impact when we have a real-time anger outburst!

By taking McClelland's study further, Rollin discovered that while feelings of anger suppress the immune system, self-induced care boosts it significantly.

It's good to know that an intentional focus on caring is more powerful than the care we feel when watching a compelling movie. But if we never focus our attention on caring, we can't consciously produce that effect. How often during the day do we make an effort to feel care? Once, twice, maybe three times? And by contrast, how often do we feel worried or anxious? More than once or twice? Worry and anxiety are the black sheep of the family of care. They're care gone awry—what researchers at the Institute call *overcare*.

# Overcare

Here's something very interesting. In Webster's dictionary, the first definitions of care are "a troubled state of mind; a suffering of mind, grief; a burdensome sense of responsibility, anxiety, concern, solicitude and worry." Those words certainly don't capture the feeling a mother has when holding her newborn baby, does it?

Webster's definition seems to have missed the first priority of care as a supportive, loving feeling. From our perspective, the burdensome state described in the dictionary definition is closer to what we define as *overcare*. When care from the heart is bombarded by niggling worries, anxieties, guesses, and estimations from the head, it can degrade from a helpful experience into a harmful one.

Overcare is one of our biggest energy deficits, and it's at the root of a lot of other unpleasant emotional states, including anxiety, fear, and depression. Overcare has many forms. Some are obvious, and others are more subtle. Overidentity, attachment, worry, and anxiety are but a few of overcare's incarnations. And while overcare in its various forms often shows up in our relationships with spouse, children, and friends, it can also tinge our relationships with things and concepts. It can, for example, take the form of overidentity with or attachment to issues, attitudes, places, things, and ideas. It can be about the environment, politics, job performance, our material possessions, our pets, our health, our future, or our past.

Because it's born from care, overcare can be hard to see. What distinguishes overcare from care is the heavy, stressful feeling that accompanies it, while true care is accompanied by a regenerative feeling. It's terribly important to care, but if we cross the line to overcare, what we feel is worrisome and stress-producing. A good question to ask ourselves is whether our care is regenerative to both the caregiver and the other recipient. If our caring intentions don't feel as if they're both adding to our energy bank account and affecting others in an uplifting way, then there's a good chance we're in overcare.

Overcare siphons off the potency of our intended care and reduces its effectiveness. Getting worried and upset doesn't help anything or anybody, even if we're worried "because we care." Problems get solved as we attain clarity and coherence, not as we worry. In fact, overcare can actually make things worse: smothering a loved one with overcare and worry tends to repulse instead of attract. Nobody likes to be nagged and worried over for too long.

Overcare is one of the main reasons people in ministerial and other care-giving professions burn out. But even those of us who are bankers and at-home moms and gardeners know what burnout feels like; at times we've all felt used up, dried up. In some institutions—many hospitals, sanitariums, hospices, and convalescent homes, for example—overcare has largely replaced true care. Why? Because the original, caring intentions of those who work in such in-stitutions—intentions born from the heart—are often drained by the un-managed mind and amalgamated with the incoherent energy of emotional discord.

It's essential that those who work with others in emotionally challenging sit-uations stay balanced in order to sustain their effectiveness. If a nurse, for in-stance, falls into the trap of overidentifying with every sick patient—taking her work home with her, worrying about those on her ward, and taking on too much responsibility for the outcome of their health dilemmas—the overcare will sap her energy.

Soon she'll feel that she has to keep a greater distance than normal from her patients to protect herself from emotional exhaustion. And yet that distance cuts her off from her heart. And without heart, she can't fully enjoy her job. She forgets why she became a nurse in the first place. That's because when she can't afford to care anymore, she doesn't feel like a caregiver.

What she doesn't realize is that there's another option—staying in her heart, continuing to care about her patients without overcare. Mother Teresa couldn't have worked all those years with some of the sickest and poorest people in the world without a huge heart that understood the difference between true care and overcare.

Jerry Kaiser, director of the Health Programs Division at HeartMath LLC, used to work with an organization that provided disaster relief for victims of hur-ricanes, floods, fires, and other catastrophic events. "When the relief teams came in," he said, "you could always tell the novices. They'd go immediately into overcare: 'Oh, no! Look at these poor people!'

"Those of us who were experienced would shake our heads. We knew that, at that level of emotional drain, these well-meaning volunteers were no good to anyone. After a day or two, they'd hit burnout and we'd have to send them home."

If we care to the point that we drain our emotional reserves, we simply don't have the energy or inclination left to care about much of anything. Overcare is the fast track to burnout. And burnout leads to no care at all.

## Eliminating Overcare

In order to eliminate the drain of overcare, we first have to become aware of the ways in which we tend to experience overcare. Everyone is different. Some of us are naturals at overidentification with factors such as physical appearance, job status, or ideas. (Yes, that's overcare too!) Others of us have overattachments to people, money, things, or issues. Under the influence of overcare in any of these guises, we're more likely to give in to worry, anxiety, anger, or fear. Pick your poison. We all have our favorites.

Luckily, listening to our heart intelligence is the best way to discover where we're expending energy in ways that aren't efficient. As we develop more of this intelligence, we'll naturally become more cognizant of our overcare.

You can start right now, if you haven't already, by making a list of your major overcares. What causes you worry and anxiety? What are you overattached to or overidentified with? Remember, overcare can be present in almost any area of your life—people, pets, things, beliefs, time pressures, or issues. It can be obvious or subtle. The overcare emotions you should be on the lookout for include anxiety, fear, depression, worry, disappointment, guilt, jealousy, and stress. All of these can range in intensity from mild to strong.

Take a few minutes to look objectively at your overcares. Write them down on the overcare inventory sheet found on page 168. This exercise isn't designed to cause you alarm. If you find yourself overcaring about your overcares, relax and shift into the area around the heart; then find a core heart feeling. Try to relieve any anxiety you have by accessing the heart.

## FREEZE-FRAMING Overcare

When you find yourself caring too much, the best thing you can do is engage your heart power and find a feeling of balanced care. This process involves taking some of the significance out of the issue and reducing the amount of emotional energy you have invested in it. As you might imagine, FREEZE-FRAME can be very useful in managing overcare. You'll learn another technique in the next chapter—CUT-THRU—that will further eliminate overcare, especially when there's a lot of energy associated with it.

Now fill out the FREEZE-FRAME worksheet on page 170—the same worksheet you responded to in Chapter 4. Pick one of the issues from your overcare

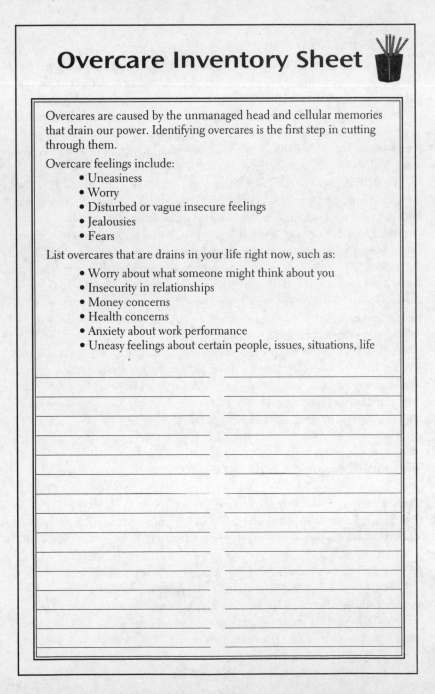

# Overcare Inventory Sheet

Overcares are caused by the unmanaged head and cellular memories that drain our power. Identifying overcares is the first step in cutting through them.

Overcare feelings include:
- Uneasiness
- Worry
- Disturbed or vague insecure feelings
- Jealousies
- Fears

List overcares that are drains in your life right now, such as:
- Worry about what someone might think about you
- Insecurity in relationships
- Money concerns
- Health concerns
- Anxiety about work performance
- Uneasy feelings about certain people, issues, situations, life

inventory sheet. Write it down under "Situation"; then, under "Head Reaction," write down a few words about how you perceive the situation and how it makes you feel.

Having set the stage, now do the FREEZE-FRAME technique and ask your heart to show you how to move from overcare back to true care; listen well, and then write down (under "Heart Intuition Response") what your heart says. Compare the before and after perspectives. See if you've determined a more efficient way to deal with your situation—one that eliminates some of your overcare and brings you back to balanced care. Most important, follow through on the advice your heart has offered you.

Don't worry: everyone experiences overcare to some degree. By identifying and then working to eliminate it, you'll be taking a major step forward. And as you continue to move ahead, you'll get to the core of what causes a lot of the hidden stress that prevents you from experiencing a more rewarding life.

## Overcare and Emotions

O vercare encompasses and gives birth to many of our least desirable emotional states. As we've seen, emotions such as disappointment, guilt, anxiety, and envy—along with many others—are often born from overcare. So are fears and insecurities, which stack up and multiply if they're not resolved. The interesting thing is that if we deal with our overcares from the heart, we eliminate a host of other emotional conditions at the same time.

Left unchecked, overcare eventually produces a low-grade angst that hangs like a cloud over every aspect of our lives. And that low-grade feeling escalates if not arrested, eventually becoming fear or even panic. Before we know it, fear starts to run the show—fear of *everything*. We can eliminate much of this emotional behavior by catching overcare early.

Since catching it requires recognizing it, let's take an in-depth look at some of the common forms overcare takes.

### Overcare in Action
#### *Generalized Anxiety and Other Fear-Based Emotions*
Let's begin with fear. Although most of us don't experience high levels of fear in our daily lives, we do feel emotions that are fundamentally fear-based, such as anxiety, worry, panic, and insecurity.

# FREEZE-FRAME Worksheet

**Here are the five steps of the FREEZE-FRAME technique:**

1. Recognize the stressful feeling, and FREEZE-FRAME it. *Take a time-out!*

2. Make a sincere effort to shift your focus away from the racing mind or disturbed emotions to the area around your heart. You can pretend that you're breathing through your heart to help focus your energy in this area. Keep your focus there for ten seconds or more.

3. Recall a positive, fun feeling or time you've had in life and attempt to re-experience it.

4. Now, using your intuition, common sense and sincerity — ask your heart, what would be a more efficient response to the situation, one that will minimize future stress?

5. Listen to what your heart says in answer to your question. It's an effective way to put your reactive mind and emotions in check — and an "in-house" source of common sense solutions!

**Situation** _____

**Head Reaction** _____

*FREEZE-FRAME*

**Heart intuition response** _____

In doing the FREEZE-FRAME exercise, I shifted from _____ to _____.

Generalized anxiety is one of the most common of these. And we often feel it for no apparent reason. But there's a reason hidden somewhere: maybe we're too concerned about a specific problem or too attached to its potential outcome. And there's a consequence as well: the habitual or ongoing experience of anxiety fosters insecurity. And left unchecked, it produces fear and panic.

Say you have a ten-year-old son who's just left for summer camp. He's never been gone for a whole week before, and although you try not to show it, you're feeling a little anxious. In your heart, you know that the camp counselors will watch out for him, but the more you think about it, the more anxious you become. After all, he's just a little boy. Without you there, he might fall out of a tree and break his neck, or drown in the lake—*anything* could happen!

When a child's safety is involved, the progression from anxiety to worry to fear to panic is a pretty quick one. But if you learn to nip anxiety in the bud, you save yourself from hours of bombardment by stressful hormones. Best of all, you avoid feeling insecure or frightened altogether.

### Performance Anxiety

More often than not, as we've seen, anxious feelings are directly associated with overcare of some kind. Performance anxiety is a perfect example. It's overcare about whether we'll meet the expectations of ourselves and others. How will we do? Will we get everything right? What are others going to think?

All of these thoughts and feelings come from overcaring about our self-image and/or overcaring about measuring up to a personal or social standard. It's important to care about doing things well, of course. But when we cross the line into overcare, our original caring is tainted by stress. It then becomes self-defeating, because it compromises our available energy to perform.

In the workplace, where competition is high, performance anxiety can reach extreme levels as people work harder and longer trying to stay ahead. Anxiety about time pressures, deadlines, communication issues, and information management is prevalent, as is anxiety about position, status, salary or benefits, raises, and performance appraisal.

Among top-level athletes, performance anxiety is such a common problem that many psychologists have built their career around the treatment of this one issue. From the snowy mountaintops of professional skiers to the playing fields of major league football stars, sports psychologists stand alongside their clients and remind them to relax, to keep their focus, to put everything else out of their mind. Their athletes know only too well that anxiety is the kiss of death for their performance.

Setting high goals is admirable, as is working hard to achieve them. But *worrying* about them is a debilitating waste of energy. It's overcare.

### Perfectionism

Perfectionism works the same way. It sets us up for inefficient emotions such as disappointment, self-judgment, and guilt. Nothing can be just good or even exceptional. It has to be *perfect*. Getting a B+ isn't good enough; you want an A. Being a successful, appreciated, well-loved wife or husband doesn't interest you; you have to be flawless. Perfectionism is overcare at its height.

Let's say you're planning a birthday party for your mother. It will soon be her eightieth birthday, and you want everything to be just right, because you always strive to be the perfect daughter. Perhaps over the years you've been taught to be perfect and you've bought into that goal, living in unconscious overcare about always hitting the highest standard.

You plan and plan for the party, overcaring as you go. Will you get the exact table you've requested at the restaurant? Will your brother, who's notorious for being late, show up on time? Will your mother have a good time? Will you receive acknowledgment for creating the perfect birthday party? You're increasingly anxious, wondering if you've attended to all the details. Everything *has* to go exactly the way you've planned it, or the party (and you) will be a failure.

Predictably, your brother is late arriving at your home. All of your overcare had no effect on his sense of punctuality. When he's only minutes late, you start to resent and judge him. Even though you drive a tad faster than the law allows, you're late getting to the restaurant, where you find that your special table has been taken. It's so typical, you think.

Your mother is fine, though, enjoying the time with her children and feeling honored that everyone cares enough to make this a special night. *She's* not in overcare about what table she sits at. But *you* feel disappointed and frustrated. Instead of having a lavish bouquet of love to offer your mother on this special birthday, you have only remnants of your loving intentions, and these are now intermingled with disappointment and resentment.

Your overcare has compromised the potency of your intended care in the name of perfectionism. And you've drained your energy. You wouldn't harm yourself that way if a little more heart security, flexibility, and emotional balance were present.

### Overattachment

Overattachment is a feeling that binds us to a person, place, object, or idea to the extent that we lose balanced perspective. A mother has a natural feeling of attachment to her child. However, if she attaches herself to the point where she can't bear to be apart from the child, her attachment promotes dependency, reinforcing her own and her child's insecurity and unhappiness.

Spouses and lovers have a natural attachment to each other. The feelings our partner kindles in us, the support and comfort he or she gives, can be tremendous assets. But if we become dependent on this attachment, we lose our own center of power. Everything the other person does (or doesn't do) becomes a source of security (or insecurity). This ill-grounded security distorts our perceptions of ourselves and of our partner. It's false security. Comparisons, jealousy, fear of loss, and actual loss are common outcomes. Relationships simply can't flourish with overcare-driven attachment.

We can also build attachments to attitudes and habits. We get in the habit of having an early-morning cup of coffee, for example, or folding the clothes a certain way, or adhering to our opinions so rigidly that we're loathe to let them go. If something interferes with our routine, we let it throw us into a "justifiable" funk. At that point, we're so set in our ways that we've lost our healthy flexibility. Yet we all know that what doesn't flex eventually breaks. Overattachment to our attitudes and routines is trouble waiting to happen.

In business, companies these days are spending millions of dollars training employees to "think out of the box." The "box" referred to in that term is made of rigid mind-sets and the inability to expand awareness. Attachment to ideas or ways of doing things limits new possibilities and can make us feel as if we're stuck in a box. A quick way out of the box can be found by developing a joint venture between the head and the heart.

Overattachment to expected outcomes or results also indicates overcare. When we add attachment to our expectancies, we set ourselves up for disappointment. If life were trying to teach us how to loosen up, this would be the perfect opportunity. The good thing about not having our expectations met is that it forces us to rethink our attachments.

As we learn to identify overcare and then make inner adjustments to recapture the feeling of true care, we remove the foundation that supports our draining emotions. That single act brings us back into balance. It's an efficient approach to emotional management, because it takes us to the source or cause of many emotional issues.

From time to time, when you're feeling emotionally out of balance, do a system check to track down any overcare that might be behind your inharmonious feelings. Once you recognize overcare in one guise or another, go to the heart and do something about it.

## The Sons and Daughters of Overcare

Worry, anxiety, and insecurity are some of the most obvious results of care running amuck. Though these feelings can sneak up on us when we least expect them, we generally know that they're there. But many subtler forms of overcare easily go unnoticed in our thought world.

Most people wouldn't think of projections, expectancies, and comparisons as overcares that need to be dealt with. These forms of mental overcare are often the culprits behind other, more noticeable unpleasant emotional conditions. In the end, they can produce large energy drains on our health and lead to breakdown. When Mark Twain said, "There's been a lot of tragedy in my life. At least half of it actually happened," he was referring to the misery that unmanaged projections can cause us.

### Projection

We use the term "projection" to describe our thoughts and mental images about the future. We all have literally thousands of thoughts about the future every day—whether it's making a shopping list for the week or planning a business meeting for next Thursday. Our long-term goals, which are invaluable for keeping our lives on track, inevitably project into the future. Hopes and dreams keep us enthusiastic about the future. But when fear and anxiety attach themselves to our projections, that's something else entirely.

Projections create untold emotional drains, but we're not usually aware of how extensive those drains are. The big deal about projections is their *cumulative* effect. Though most of us don't recognize projections as problems—after all, *everybody* projects into the future—drop by drop they leach away the energy we need to create a positive future. As a result, we don't have enough energy to experience "quality" in our life. Everything may seem okay on the surface, but something's still missing.

If we walk across the desert with water in a bucket full of holes, we're not going to have anything left to drink when we need it. The more holes, the faster the water is depleted; but even one hole would drain the water out. That one hole could be a projection that drains the bucket in fifteen steps or in three miles.

Most of us have low-grade projections operating constantly all day long. Even if individually they seem like no big deal—each one just a pinhole hole in our bucket—remember that it takes only one leak to drain that bucket dry.

It's just physics: energy has to be accounted for. When we extend our fears and insecurities by projecting them into the future, we encourage more fears to rush in, creating an even greater energy drain. If we believe in those fears, we actually help create what we most fear.

Think about it. How much energy is spent wondering about how things will work out? How often do we project that we won't have enough time, won't meet an important deadline, or won't be able to communicate with someone? How much are those projections and overcares costing us? The energy drains they initiate won't stop themselves. It's up to us to notice and stop them.

Have you ever left the house on a trip and started worrying, after you were miles from home, about whether or not you turned off the oven? You're almost certain you did, but what if . . . ? If you have reason to think you really might have left the oven on, then taking action is an appropriate response. Stop at your first opportunity and call to have a neighbor check it out. That's natural and responsible. But if you're picturing your entire house burning down on the basis of an unsubstantiated what-if, you're in overcare projection. And all that fretting and worrying will register as a deficit on your inner asset/deficit balance sheet.

We can also experience projections around long-term issues such as finding fulfillment or success, meeting the right mate, getting the right job, raising well-adjusted children, and so on. Considering our future is in and of itself very appropriate—but not if that consideration turns into overcare, producing a fearful wondering about future security for ourselves and others. That kind of projection doesn't serve us or anybody else well.

Here's another interesting example. We like to call it "high-speed projection." Have you ever found yourself saying, "Life sure is going well. I wonder when that's going to end and things are going to change for the worse?"

Right in the middle of good times, with no reality-based reason, we can sabotage our well-being by overcaring and projecting about what might happen. The thoughts and feelings of pending disaster fly through our minds at high speed. We don't even know what hit us. Without realizing it, our speculation has inhibited our ability to be as fully appreciative of our current situation as we could (and should) be.

And what about idealistic projections? We imagine a glorious new career or wonderful vacation and invest our hopes and identity in that, then end up devastated if the reality doesn't match the projection.

Projecting outcomes is automatic in most people. In fact, everyone does it, though to different degrees. It's not bad, but it's wise to learn how to manage your projections.

Since the thoughts and feelings of projection can be subtle, ask your heart to help you see them. Try not to identify with them as you observe them. Go to neutral and let your heart intelligence show you a different perspective. It takes a fine-tuned level of emotional management to stop projections as they arise. Then appreciate your life without worrying or projecting a future reality that may or may not actually happen.

### Expectancy

We generally take it for granted that we'll be treated with respect and good manners by our family, our co-workers, even our waiter at a restaurant. Whether people actually treat us that way or not, we all have expectations. We also expect predictable results from our efforts. We expect meetings to take place on schedule. We expect people to do what they say they will. And when things go wrong, we feel entitled to the stress we feel. And all too often—in all these many ways—expectancy leads us around by the nose.

When we care too much about life's conforming to our expectations, we're setting ourselves up for disappointment. As we all know, life just isn't that compliant. Reality will eventually—and often—fail to meet our expectations. The disappointment we feel can lead to despair, which can then become depression. We feel like victims. All of this takes a toll on our bodies and negatively impacts our longevity.

Expectancy also leads to blame, which consumes a lot of energy and doesn't fix anything. It just makes things continually worse. Blame drains the blamer. It's not the thoughts of blame that cause the heaviest drain, though; it's the significance and emotional energy that go into supporting the blame.

Years ago, when I (Doc) got out of school, I took a job at a furniture factory. One day my car broke down and for a period of many weeks I would need a ride to get to work.

A friend agreed to give me a ride regularly if I met him halfway down the road between our houses. Things went well for a couple of weeks. I was glad I could count on him while my car was being fixed.

One morning it was raining as I trudged down that dirt road to meet my ride. I stood expectantly, getting wetter and wetter, as I waited for my friend. He never showed up, though he knew I was depending on him. I couldn't believe it. I was so disappointed that I couldn't think straight.

After unsuccessfully trying to hitchhike, I finally knocked on a stranger's door, dripping wet, and called a cab. And I decided to take a cab from then on. I left him a message to that effect but offered no explanation.

When I finally got my car back, I ran into my friend and unloaded on him.

Nothing I said had to do with my appreciation for the fact that he'd indeed picked me up without fail for a time before letting me down.

He said he'd tried to call me that rainy morning to explain that he'd had a flat tire. Eager to make things right between us, he even showed me the receipt for the new tire. I quickly realized how foolish I'd been to hold a grudge against him for so long. I almost lost a good friend because my idealistic expectations weren't tempered by a consideration of life's unexpected occurrences.

It's odd when you think of how idealistic our expectations can be. They're fantasies about the way we'd like life to work, nothing more. We can't control how everything will turn out. And even when everything goes right, sometimes we mess things up ourselves. How can we hold others to a higher standard than ourselves?

The positive power of expectancy is found through the heart. But that power is only as positive as your ability to release your expectation if it isn't fulfilled, take on a new, more realistic perspective, and cut your losses.

### Comparison

In this context, *comparison* means measuring ourselves against others—assessing who we are (self-image) and what we have versus who someone else is and what she has.

Comparisons that cause emotional stress arise out of our own insecurities and frailties. For example, we can overcare about whether we're as smart or as beautiful as someone else and lose sight of our own good qualities. We can envy other people's acquisitions and achievements—their cars, their families, their houses, their jobs—and completely miss how happy we could be in our own lives if we'd stop comparing. Feeling this sort of comparison is very different from having successful role models or a healthy admiration for other people.

Status is a common comparative playground. "Do I have as much [money, prestige, you name it] as he does?" "Is our son going to get into as good a college as our neighbor's daughter?" "Don't I deserve the corner office just as much as my colleague does?" "Isn't my job as important as my friend's?" All these questions reveal overcare about what we have versus what others have.

If we've taken an honest inventory from the heart in the previous exercises, we may now be feeling that we have more than we thought we did. Still, though, we always want more (and feel *entitled* to more). That's due in part to a natural urge for growth and fulfillment, but comparisons make us lose perspective and choke appreciation for all that we *do* have.

A mutual friend inherited a substantial amount of property, stocks, and personal belongings when his mother died. His brother received an inheritance of equal value, but he was also given their mother's diamond wedding ring. When he found out about it, our friend went into extreme overcare. He started obsessing about why his brother got the ring. It had been so important to their mother, he said. Did this mean she loved his brother more? Working himself up into a frenzy, he began questioning everything about their inheritance, trying to second-guess their mother's decisions: "Why did I get the house while my brother got the farm? Is the farm better? What was she trying to say?"

With overcare coloring his perspective, our friend saw every innocent line in the will, every generous bequest, as a potential source of pain. After many miserable weeks, he gradually let go of his perceptions and made peace with his mother's decisions. He realized that he didn't really doubt her love for him and that he had, in fact, received a wonderful inheritance, ring or not.

If comparison runs away with us, it leads to envy and jealousy—fertile ground for other deficit emotions, such as blame, resentment, and even hate. Think about it. We can start out caring about something or someone and, because of a single jealous thought, end up resenting or even hating that thing or person. That's the potential of unmanaged overcare.

With overcare, the focus is on what we *don't have* in comparison to others. Overcare not only reduces appreciation of what we do have but also seriously lowers our self-appreciation and self-esteem. The solution, of course, is to develop a stronger sense of inner security. Heart intelligence helps build security, but it won't happen overnight.

If you're in the habit of making unfavorable comparisons between yourself and others, you're in the habit of being too hard on yourself. It's just not possible that you're worse at everything than everyone you know. So it's important that, from the moment you decide to work on this element of comparison overcare, you lighten up. Give yourself some self-care. The best way to stop making comparisons is little by little. Realize that a lot of our overcares come from social programming in our families, schools, and society. Appreciate yourself for improvements as you go instead of expecting instant success.

## Tackling Projection, Expectancy, and Comparison

When we check projection, expectancy, and comparison at the door, balancing our overcares with the wisdom and care of the heart, we leave room for human frailties and for life to be life. We realize that growing up emotionally entails not expecting everything to meet our expectations. That realization helps us sincerely care about things without slipping into overcare, which means we don't have to go through the stress that overcare creates.

Here are five tips that can help to eliminate projection, expectancy, and comparison:

1. Become observant of your thoughts and feelings and make a sincere effort to see where you might be prone to regularly experiencing overcare.

2. When you find yourself experiencing unhealthy projection, expectancy, or comparison, remember that those energy deficits are draining your energy reserves. That perspective will give you the motivation needed to move beyond them.

3. Try to take some of the significance out of projective, expectant, and comparative thoughts and feelings. They're usually not as important as they seem.

4. When you find yourself experiencing any of these overcares, make an effort to stop, do a short FREEZE-FRAME, and ask your heart to show you how to transform each overcare into true care. Making contact with your heart intelligence will allow you to see things in a more comprehensive way and give new direction for your care.

5. Activate the core heart feeling of appreciation. Appreciate the way things are instead of overidentifying with a situation or issue, and appreciate yourself for having the awareness to catch these subtle overcares.

Learning to care more for yourself and others isn't about being flawless and never experiencing overcare. It's neither an instant nor a finite process. It takes time to weed overcare out of your life, and the process is ongoing, but it's actually fun to start looking for overcare and freeing yourself from it.

As your heart intelligence becomes more readily accessible, you won't have to be on the lookout for every stray thought or feeling. The signals from the heart will be clearer, letting you know without prompting when your care has become overcare. Every time you eliminate an overcare, the relief will be tremendous, and you'll store away power that will make dealing with overcare easier the next time.

Soon you'll discover for yourself that transmuting overcare into true care is one of the most rewarding and regenerative accomplishments you can experience. Eliminating overcare is an act of self-care that will enhance your life in ways you've never imagined. It will also enhance your ability to intelligently care for the people and social issues that are important to you.

Often, when we're giving a seminar, we talk about cultivating self-care. Most participants love the concept—and why not? Just the idea feels nurturing and good to our souls. Most of us were taught to give ourselves the short end of the stick. Setting aside time to care for ourselves seems like a luxury.

Because of inexperience, the first things that come to mind around self-care are fairly simple. "Hugging my puppy makes me feel so good that I'll do it more often!" a student might say. Or "I know: I'll light some candles and take a long, hot bath." Great suggestions. But self-care goes much deeper than that.

Caring for yourself enough to generate love for yourself throughout the day—for no reason at all (except that you're worth it!)—sends a strong message to your heart. Once it knows what you're up to, it will begin to help you generate that love. This isn't narcissism; it's self-health. Eliminating overcare and other energy drains is most quickly and painlessly accomplished by stepping back from the clatter of the mind and letting yourself be motivated by a deep sense of self-care. With self-care, you'll begin to amplify your capacity to care until it naturally flows out from you to yourself, your loved ones, and the world around you.

## A Return to Care

Care is a valuable and vital resource, far more precious than people realize. It revitalizes you and acts as a soothing tonic for the human system.

Yet people squander their care in overcare, then burn out and end up with no care at all. Many personal, interpersonal, and social problems will be solved as humanity develops a more mature sense of care. At the deepest level, it's real love and care that people crave. Give those things, and you'll receive them. Through your caring deeds and actions, you'll truly make your mark on the world.

It's not care, but overcare, that stops most people from caring. Overcares will come and go, but it's important to remember that we have to care in the first place to get into overcare. It's about balance, about walking a fine line. And the heart can give us that balance, allowing us to express our care without letting its regenerating warmth and reassuring power slip away.

In today's culture, unconscious overcare for ourselves and issues is so rampant that it's become a social disease. It spawns stress in mega-doses, creating so much incoherence in people and society that it ranks at the top of the list of human energy drains. The importance of eliminating this stressor can't be stated too strongly.

Care paves the way for intuition. Overcare then comes along and eats up the pavement, leaving us without a road to travel on. That's why we don't get anywhere. Care provides a conduit for our spirit's expression in the midst of our social existence. The more we truly care, the more we'll come to know ourselves and others. Care provides the key to unlocking our potential and making it real. The bridge between all that we can be and all that we are lies in the heart. There we can find the bridge of care clearly marked.

## KEY POINTS TO REMEMBER

➤ Care is a powerful motivator. It inspires and gently reassures us. Care *feels* good—whether we're giving or receiving it.

➤ Research shows that feelings of care boost the immune system, while feelings of anger suppress it significantly.

➤ When care from the heart is bombarded by worries and anxieties, projections and expectations, it degrades into overcare.

➤ Overcare siphons off the potency of our intended care and reduces its effectiveness. Problems get solved as we attain more clarity and coherence, not through worry.

➤ Thousands suffer from overcare-driven exhaustion and burnout. They feel that they've cared too much and can't care any more.

➤ Overcare that's left unchecked eventually produces a low-grade angst that hangs like a cloud over your entire life.

➤ Signals from the heart let you know when your care has become overcare, if you're willing to listen. Every time you eliminate an overcare, the relief is tremendous, and you store away power that makes fighting overcare easier the next time.

➤ By identifying and then working to eliminate overcare, you approach the core of what causes a lot of the hidden stress that prevents you from experiencing a more rewarding life. Eliminating overcare is an act of self-care that will enhance your life in ways you've never imagined.

➤ Care provides a conduit for your spirit's expression in the midst of human existence. The more you truly care, the more you'll come to know of yourself and others.

➤ A return to care is at the top of the list when it comes to societal need.

# CHAPTER 9

# Cut-Thru to Emotional Maturity

As the president of a high-tech computer company in Omaha, Carol McDonald handles more high-stress situations in a week than many people face all year. She loves the challenge of overcoming obstacles, and she clearly does it well. But when she got the news that her alcoholic father was in desperate need of intervention, her emotional balance was tested.

"We found him under the bed, curled fetally and drenched in his own urine. His eyes were blackened underneath, nose and temple lacerated due to falling against the bathroom vanity, dead-weighted in drunkenness. He was wailing, screaming in flashbacks from terrible times past that even two and a half bottles of scotch couldn't blot out. He was gray and bloated beyond his seventy-five years, not so much by age as by alcohol. And he'd had lots of it over the decades, until it began to eat up his brain in atrophy and dementia. I suppose in its own way, the anesthetic finally worked.

"My husband and I swooped in and moved him across the country and into our home, paving the way for him to find the will to attempt detox treatment. This process was gradual indeed, for one can't take a chronic alcoholic and deprive him of his alcohol until medical supervision intervenes. Instead, you meter out his liquid fixes by monitoring the intake, hoping for the best. That is, until a treatment center relieves you with an opening so that the real healing can begin.

"Although we hid the bottle, he'd still find it sometimes, so I'd return home from work to find him sloshed and silly, oblivious and vacant—a shell of the human being who once glued my entire world together.

"I got angry. And resentful. And judgmental of his pathetic display. Over time I began to care too much, suffocating from worry over a situation that was growing bigger than my ability to fix it. When my judgment and anger started to choke and strangle my compassion, I'd go to our patio and practice the CUT-THRU technique, sometimes over and over, until the anxiety passed right through my body, like the wind breezing through a screen door.

"During his summer stay, the effectiveness of CUT-THRU allowed me to provide my father with the love and support he needed day by day and moment to moment. The power of my heart rippled through both my mind and my body, recalibrating my sincere acceptance of him and sustaining my care without killing myself with overcare. I know in my heart that CUT-THRU has been a life-saving tool."

By sincerely applying the CUT-THRU technique, Carol was able to manage her emotions, reduce overcare, and experience an extraordinary shift within herself. She was caught up in a situation that offered many opportunities to experience a host of justified emotions, but she knew in her heart that she couldn't live like that. She looked to the power of her heart to gain release—and she found it.

## What Is CUT-THRU?

The purpose of CUT-THRU is to help people recognize and reprogram the subconscious emotional memory paths that, through long-term reinforcement, influence our perception, color our day-to-day thoughts and feelings, and condition our responses to future situations.

Scientists have found that emotional circuitry is susceptible to enhancement in much the same way as any other memory trace. [1] The CUT-THRU technique provides a reliable method to move out emotions that aren't to your liking, enhance emotions you do want, and change your neural architecture. That covers a lot of territory. If you're like most people, there are many feelings you could do without and others you wish you could experience more often. Emotional management is a key to shifting into a new dimension of emotional freedom, and it's a necessity if you're wanting new levels of awareness and inner security.

As we've pointed out, emotions are very complex and our emotional patterning can be hard to change. FREEZE-FRAME provides a reliable tool for managing many emotions and emotional reactions. Sometimes, however, when we FREEZE-FRAME we can see clearly how to better deal with a situation but we don't feel completely released emotionally. For deeply ingrained emotional issues, it takes more than doing a one-minute technique such as FREEZE-FRAME to move beyond them; it takes going deeper into the realm of heart intelligence — and that's when we need CUT-THRU.

We're all familiar with the term "cut through," meaning "get to the heart of the matter." Perhaps you've had the experience of working with a group to solve a problem. After the discussion goes around and around without resolution, someone finally says, "Okay, let's just cut through all the irrelevant stuff and get back to the real issue." Stopping to focus again on the main point allows things to get back on track.

It's like the story in Greek mythology about the Gordian knot. They say that Gordius, King of Phrygia, once tied a knot so entwined that no one could untie it. Then he staked everything on that knot, claiming that if anyone could release it, he'd make that person ruler of all Asia.

The idea appealed to Alexander the Great, who was very much interested in being the ruler of Asia. Why wage a battle with thousands of men when he could simply outsmart a king? After taking one look at the knot, Alexander surmised that it couldn't be untied. But he didn't see that as a problem. He pulled out his sword and with one clean stroke cut through the Gordian knot, thereby becoming the ruler of all Asia.

Trying to untangle your emotions can be like struggling to untie a knot. Sometimes the struggle only makes it worse. CUT-THRU is designed to help you cut through the Gordian knot of your emotions. It allows you to move more quickly through emotional distortion to a place of resolution.

In the process, you let go of your personal grudges and perspectives, of the need to wallow in your feelings. It's not that you don't feel them; you do. But you force yourself to transcend them. You make a choice that takes you to the next level of emotional management.

Think of the extent to which little children are at the mercy of their emotions. Take a toy from a toddler, and she bursts into tears, overwhelmed with disappointment. As children physically mature, they develop new options that give them more control over their emotions. Soon they realize that they can ask for the toy back or simply get up and get it themselves. Knowing that they can get results allows older children to stave off the feeling of distress at least long enough to take action.

Most of us stop at that level. We learn a certain amount of emotional management in the natural course of physical development, and we make do with that. But with the right tools, you can manage your emotions deliberately and effectively. Instead of straining to hold off an emotion while you figure out what to do, or endlessly trying to untangle a mess of emotions to get to the crux of a problem, you can learn to shift out of emotional turbulence into an emotional coherence that's balanced, peaceful, and clear. You achieve emotional coherence through heart coherence—a balanced state achieved when your emotions come into alignment with your deep heart. With that kind of clarity, a workable solution to your problem often comes quickly.

CUT-THRU facilitates emotional coherence. It allows you to transform the emotions that are tangling you up and causing you stress into feelings of peace and regeneration. And it does that without resorting to rationalization or repression.

Though the Institute's evidence proves that this is a powerful, effective technique, it's important to realize that it's not magic. A name like "CUT-THRU" might lead you to imagine that it's an instant formula for whisking away troubling emotions. That's not always the case.

Although anyone can use CUT-THRU to help clear the way through an emotional jungle, it's not another pie-in-the-sky self-help technique. If you're honest with yourself, you know that your emotions are terribly difficult to manage. As human beings, we've cultivated our minds but have neglected our emotions. Even the greatest intellects have often left their emotions to chance, not bothering to consciously lead themselves toward the emotional management that would have made their lives so much easier and less frustrating.

As you begin the process, you'll discover that some emotions can be shifted very quickly, while others—generally those with a longer emotional history—take more time. Keep in mind that negative emotional patterns that have been reinforced for years (or even decades) have created well-worn neural pathways through your brain. If you stop traveling down those pathways, they'll soon give way to the new patterns you're creating, but it takes repetition. You can rest assured that your physiology will respond to your intervention.

Used properly, CUT-THRU can yield significantly greater emotional management. But achieving any real depth with this technique requires sincere application and mature contemplation. Read through the detailed descriptions of the attitude and emotional shifts intended with each step; then go back and practice the steps. It's worth taking the time to explore each aspect of CUT-THRU carefully.

# The Six Steps of CUT-THRU

1.  Be Aware of how you Feel about the issue at hand.

2.  Focus in the Heart and Solar Plexus—Breathe love and appreciation through this area for ten seconds or more to help anchor your attention there.

3.  Assume Objectivity about the feeling or issue—as if it were someone else's problem.

4.  Rest in Neutral—in your Rational, Mature Heart.

5.  Soak and Relax any disturbed or perplexing feelings in the compassion of the heart, Dissolving the Significance a little at a time. Take your time doing this step; there's no time limit. Remember, it's not the problem that causes energy drain as much as the significance you assign to the problem.

6.  After Extracting as much Significance as you can, from your Deep Heart sincerely Ask for appropriate guidance or insight. If you don't get an answer, Find something to Appreciate for awhile. Appreciation of anything often facilitates intuitive clarity on issues you've been working on.

Repeat steps as needed. Some issues require more time than others soaking in the heart to mature into new understanding and release.

You may have noticed that some of the language in these steps is more abstract than that used in describing FREEZE-FRAME. Because CUT-THRU deals with a very complex process—transforming deeply stored, incoherent emotional patterns into heart coherence—it can't be expressed as simply. The words used here were very carefully chosen to help you achieve the attitude and emotional shifts needed. Notice that the first letter of some of the words is capitalized. These are key words for each step.

Once you've practiced CUT-THRU a few times, you'll better understand the mechanics. With that deeper understanding, you'll find the steps simpler to follow; and you'll be able to move from step to step using only the key words (or perhaps simple buzzwords that you create). That simplification will make the steps easier to remember.

Now let's take a detailed look at each step.

## Step 1

*Be Aware of how you Feel about the issue at hand.*

It seems self-evident that we'd know how we feel about an issue. And often we do: there are many times when we're upset, worried, anxious, or overwhelmed and we know it. But we're much less in touch with our feelings than we think. It's very common to shove aside feelings that are draining us or to get so caught up in a feeling that we don't recognize it for what it is.

Maybe you get up on the wrong side of the bed and have some cross words with your spouse. That upsets you, but after a few minutes the intensity of the incident decreases. Still, as you go on about your business, the feeling lingers. You're edgy and out of sorts for hours. Although you don't stop to realize that those cross words have set up an emotional imbalance, you experience a steady emotional drain that colors the rest of your day.

From that diminished state, things start to get fuzzy. Someone in the office does something wrong, and you really let him have it. Yet if you were to stop and be aware of how you really feel about his mistake, you'd realize that you don't feel strongly at all. *Anyone* might have made the same mistake. What you're *really* reacting to is the earlier fight with your spouse (and the crankiness you felt even before that).

Sometimes we feel something slightly unpleasant, but because it's so subtle, we just accept it; we don't do anything about it. Overcare is a good example. We rarely notice when we cross that line from genuine concern into a draining, counterproductive state of overcare. Intellectually, it's a tricky distinction that varies from person to person. But from the heart's perspective, it's not so hard to figure out: overcare doesn't *feel* good. You can learn to recognize that worried feeling and CUT-THRU to balanced care on the spot.

Like overcare, long-standing issues can keep you in emotional turmoil. Lingering resentments, unresolved feelings of guilt, or other old emotional wounds are constant energy drains that need to be addressed if you want to get the most out of life.

When any issue comes up, past or present, learn to observe your feelings more closely. If you're not feeling emotionally balanced, it's time to realize that you can make a shift to a more peaceful and beneficial emotional state—and then initiate that shift. Of course, you can try FREEZE-FRAME first. That technique is very useful for bringing your emotions into balance, and you'll be surprised at how effective it can be at stopping emotional and mental drains. If you don't feel a significant emotional shift after doing a FREEZE-FRAME in any given situation, however, begin practicing the steps of CUT-THRU.

## Step 2

*Focus in the Heart and Solar Plexus—Breathe love and appreciation through this area for ten seconds or more to help anchor your attention there.*

In this step, you'll breathe slowly through the region of your body that extends from your chest down to your stomach, or gut. Imagine that your breath is going in and out through this area of your body. Feeling love and appreciation as you breathe helps create coherence. Your solar plexus is just below the sternum, where your diaphragm connects to the other muscles in your chest. Great opera singers and other stage performers learn to breathe through their solar plexus to give them a deep boost of power to project their voices.

Step 2 begins a process of calming your emotions so that you can gain more balance and stability. Breathing through the area of the heart and solar plexus will help to keep your emotional energies focused and grounded.

Often we feel strong emotions in the solar plexus. We now understand why: it contains those ever-important neurons and neurotransmitters. Like the heart, it has its own little brain. Strong emotions impact this little brain, which explains why we feel nervousness as a knot in the stomach when we're anxious or upset.

In a 1996 *New York Times* article, Dr. Michael Gershon, a professor of anatomy and cell biology at Columbia-Presbyterian Medical Center in New York, said, "When the central brain encounters a frightening situation, it releases stress hormones that prepare the body to fight or flee. The stomach contains many sensory nerves that are stimulated by this chemical surge—hence the butterflies."

It's also believed that the nervous system in the solar plexus communicates directly with the lower brain centers activating some of our more primal instincts—thus the term "gut reaction." Dr. Gershon says, "Just as the central brain affects the gut, the gut brain can talk back to the head." Dr. David Wingate, professor of gastrointestinal science at the University of London and consultant at the Royal London Hospital, adds, "Most gut sensations that enter conscious awareness are negative things like pain and bloatedness. We don't expect to feel anything good from the gut, but that doesn't mean signals are absent." [2]

Now remember, the heart is by far the strongest source of rhythmic bioelectricity in your body. It's your most dominant biological oscillator, and its powerful rhythms can pull the other biological oscillators into entrainment. By concentrating on both the heart and the solar plexus as you breathe love and appreciation, you're aligning the brain in the gut with the brain in the heart. The heart will automatically harmonize the communication between them.

You'll find that this interplay between heart, solar plexus, and brain gives you a more anchored feeling. Instead of drifting on a sea of emotions, you'll feel more fixed. A ship can float a little bit in one direction or another when it's anchored, but it can't get far from the place where the anchor was let down. The result is a secure, stable feeling.

Anchoring sets up a new reference point, meaning that when you're out of phase emotionally, you won't have to be out as long before getting back to emotional balance, or try as hard to get there. As you become anchored, you'll feel more buoyant. More power and coherence will flow through your system. This will give you more capacity to move beyond emotional distortion.

## Step 3

*Assume Objectivity about the feeling or issue—as if it were someone else's problem.*

When you're caught up in the emotions surrounding an issue, you can't be objective. How many irrational and damaging decisions have you made while so swamped with emotions that the bigger picture was completely lost?

Without objectivity, an issue can seem larger than it is, causing increased emotional reactivity and overidentity. Most emotional issues are due to overidentity in the first place; in other words, your head plunges into a reaction ahead of your heart. The more emotional you get, the less objective you become. The less objective you are, the more emotional you become; and the cycle continues until you run out of emotional energy, break down in tears, or blow up. Then you have to pick up the pieces. In order to free yourself from the whirlwind of emotions, you have to break this cycle at some point in the process.

Marriage counselors and mediators in disputes spend about 80 percent of their time trying to get the opponents to step back and see things more objectively. Only about 20 percent of their time is spent on specific solutions. The solutions are there, waiting to be selected and implemented, when the parties are willing to compromise. But they can't even consider a compromise while they're busy blaming each other and trying to win an argument.

The same is true when you're mediating a dispute between you and yourself. You'll never get anywhere if your mind is made up. If you're determined to blame someone or to be right at any cost, there's no way to see things objectively. The old saying, "Don't confuse me with the facts; my mind is made up" comes out of just this situation. And we've all been there. As long as we maintain a vested interest in the outcome, we're too personally involved to be impartial.

"Assuming objectivity" means finding the integrity to *disengage* from the feeling or issue that's troubling you. But putting yourself in a disengagement chamber isn't easy. In fact, Step 3 can be the most challenging step, especially if the problem is emotionally charged. "If I feel resistance and can't pull my energy out of the emotion," one person said, "then I send in a white flag and suspend it from the heart."

Remember those old cowboy and Indian movies you loved as a child? The cowboys with their covered wagons and roaming kids are on one side of the hill, and the Indians on their horses are on the other, ready for battle. You've gotten to know the characters, so you're at the edge of your seat, hoping for some heart so that no one gets killed. Then one side throws out a white flag and you feel the suspension of tension. There's a chance for heart negotiation as they suspend their emotions for awhile and come to a compromise. As in those movies, suspending your feelings for awhile so that you can address them objectively in the midst of emotional turmoil can save the day.

Learning to "disidentify"—to observe ourselves as if we were someone else—is one of the key elements for success in gestalt therapy. But if we're really steamed up and identified with an issue, stepping back is the last thing the mind wants to do. We've got a point to make, right? And in the heat of the moment, it seems like making that point is the most important thing in the world—no matter how many times we've made it before: "Life isn't fair!" or "People are insensitive!" or "She does that every time!" You'd think we'd be bored with the repetition, but we're not.

The next time you catch yourself appropriating an issue, try Step 3 instead. Tell yourself that you're going to disengage from the issue; then throw out a white flag and attempt to observe the feelings or issue as someone else's problem. Pretend that you're watching another person deal with this—not you. How does this scene look from a distance? The perception shift can be amazing.

It's remarkable what good advice we can give to other people. We sound amazingly mature and objective when it's *their* problem instead of *ours*. As you attempt to carry out Step 3 on a particular issue, think about how you'd advise that hypothetical someone else who's in your shoes. How would you suggest that he or she handle the situation? Is the emotional reaction you're witnessing appropriate? Does the person really need to feel that way?

In Step 3 you make an effort to step off the stage and observe what's going on. You become a member of the audience instead of the lead actor. You may be surprised at what good advice you have for yourself once you're clear of your emotional attachment.

Assuming objectivity allows you to become less identified with the issue, which reduces the amount of emotional energy you have invested in it. By greatly reducing the burden of significance you place on the problem, you begin to regain emotional coherence.

## Step 4

*Rest in Neutral—in your Rational, Mature Heart.*

Once Step 3 carries you to a point of relative objectivity, you become more neutral and begin to experience a rational and mature emotional response to the issue at hand—a response that's based on heart intelligence.

As we've seen, a neutral state provides an opportunity for new possibilities to emerge. Remember, going into neutral doesn't mean that you have to accept or buy into anything. It's an impartial state that allows for new probabilities. If you can find a neutral place to rest during an emotional storm, you'll quickly shift your attitudes and feelings. And that shift will be actual, not perceptual. In other words, you won't simply make a mental shift, but you'll experience distinctly different attitudes and feelings as you surrender your mind to your deep heart. In this CUT-THRU step, relax in neutral, find some peace, and make contact with your heart intelligence.

Your "rational, mature heart" is that deep place inside your heart that's more reasonable in its assessments. This aspect of your heart intelligence provides perspectives and feelings that allow you to consider what's best for your well-being. It provides understanding that makes it easier to shift your attitude and find more balanced, regenerative feelings.

Many of the most effective therapeutic approaches used today involve what's called "cognitive restructuring"—that is, redirecting thoughts to interpret life's events in a more realistic and positive way. Research at the Institute suggests that the heart has to be engaged if a cognitive shift is to take place; otherwise, cognitive restructuring can be an intellectual exercise that has little power to shift the emotions.

The rational, mature heart offers new direction that can help to retrain the mind, encouraging it to let go of inflexible attitudes that confine your ability to make emotional shifts. From the deep heart you can see what needs to change—and why.

In the middle of an episode of emotional tension, you've probably longed for the ability and the poise to smooth out your feelings. That longing is the voice of the heart telling you that something needs to be balanced. Though you hear the voice, you may remain stuck in emotional dissonance. In the next two steps of the CUT-THRU technique, you can reestablish your poise and emotional coherence. Steps 1 through 4 have prepared you for the last phase of the technique, which helps you clear out any remaining disturbed or dissonant feelings.

## Step 5

*Soak and Relax any disturbed or perplexing feelings in the compassion of the heart, Dissolving the Significance a little at a time. Take your time doing this step; there's no time limit. Remember, it's not the problem that causes energy drain as much as the significance you assign to the problem.*

As we saw in an earlier chapter, emotions are energy in motion. Remember that when you feel upset about something, it's not the actual issue that's causing discomfort. It's the significance you've placed on the issue. As Nietzsche said, "There are no facts, only interpretations." Everything upsetting about a given issue has been added by your interpretation, which is totally subjective. Someone looking at things from a different point of view might draw completely different conclusions.

You can let go of the significance without fear that you're letting go of the "truth" about the issue. What you're releasing isn't the truth. It's nothing but incoherent energy reinforced by a belief in its significance. That's what makes up disturbed feelings.

In Step 5 you use the coherent power of the heart to take out the weight or energy you've invested in the issue, thereby reducing its significance. By doing Steps 1 through 4, you've accessed your deeper heart and are now prepared to clean out the emotional residue. Let the power of the heart do the rest of the work for you.

Focus in the area around your heart and take uncomfortable or disturbed feelings into the heart, soaking them there to dissolve the significance. Though the language is necessarily abstract, this step isn't hard to do. All it requires is letting go of your identity with the emotions you're feeling and then soaking in the coherent energy of the heart. Feeling compassion as you do this helps increase coherence.

You know plenty about soaking—whether it's dirty dishes, stained clothes, or grubby silverware. If you soak a stubborn stain overnight in a solvent, you make the actual cleaning job a lot easier, because the initial density of the stain has been taken out. Maybe you'll still have to scrub it and run it through a wash cycle, or treat it with some fabric softener. But by then much of the resistant stain or stiffness is gone.

Your emotional problems can be dealt with in the same way when approached from the heart. Your heart regulates the flow of your blood, but it will also regulate the flow of your emotions if you let it. You just have to be sincere and realize that your heart—your own built-in source of self-security and inner nourishment—can help you take the significance and accumulation out of emotional issues. Often it's old, unconscious identities that keep you feeling stuck. You may not even know what they are. In Step 5 you use the power of the heart to dissipate and transmute unpleasant emotional energy. You soak it in the solvent of the heart—in your love and compassion—then ease the disturbance out.

When Carol McDonald practiced CUT-THRU to deal with the emotional drain of helping her father, she had the sensation that "the anxiety passed right through [her] body, like the wind breezing through a screen door." Soaking feelings such as worry, anger, anxiety, and overcare in the heart reduces their density. Once the resistance of that density is gone, you can process even subtle feelings of tension through the heart; more important, the caring feelings of the heart can flow through you easily, and a feeling of lightness and clarity follows.

Take your time with this step. As you relax and soak in the heart, a lot of important work can get done. Most old patterns are deeply etched in your neural circuitry, as we've seen. Depending on how you're feeling in the moment, and how deep and well-reinforced the old feelings are, you may have a lot of emotional energy to release. If so, give yourself a little extra compassion and self-care; allow your inner systems to rest. As you soak, don't worry about trying to feel love or care, about getting an answer, about whether you're doing the technique right, or about anything of that nature. Just try to let out the uncomfortable feelings in the warmth of the heart, until you feel a release. Ease them out softly and delicately and let the coherence of the heart work for you.

Soaking in the heart won't always make an issue disappear. However, if your effort is sincere, the process takes enough of the density out of your cellular memory that you can address the issue more intelligently when you return to it. Furthermore, the issue won't be nearly as overpowering.

## Step 6

*After Extracting as much Significance as you can, from your Deep Heart sincerely Ask for appropriate guidance or insight. If you don't get an answer, Find something to Appreciate for awhile. Appreciation of anything often facilitates intuitive clarity on issues you've been working on.*

Now, having used the heart to release old and uncomfortable feelings, you'll be able to more easily hear the intuitive voice of your heart intelligence. Sincerely ask your heart for new understanding and direction. But do so with maturity, realizing that the heart won't flash an answer on a neon sign. When you apply the steps of CUT-THRU or FREEZE-FRAME, you won't always get an answer right away—or even in an hour or two. Sometimes the answer shows up the next day or even the next week. You have to allow time for things to play out.

A lot of the time the heart answers through delicate intuitive feelings or subtle understanding. It can also answer loud and clear, however. Respect both types of response and have the awareness to know that the process of learning to listen to the heart takes time.

If you don't get an answer right away, take what clarity and release you've gained from doing Steps 1 through 6 and use them to find something to appreciate. There are several reasons for this. First, appreciation is such a powerful core heart feeling that it can help complete the release of disturbed feelings. Second, activating a feeling of appreciation can help you shift your attitude quickly and keep you from falling back into emotional identity with your issue. Third, feeling appreciation for awhile often activates intuitive clarity on other issues you're working on. So try to find something, anything, to appreciate until you get clear direction from your heart. Then, when that direction comes, follow it.

Repeat the steps of Cut-Thru as needed. Some emotions can be cut through quickly; others take time and repetition. If the same unpleasant feelings keep coming up, hold onto your patience and try again—and again. Remember, some patterns have been reinforced for years, so don't expect them to disappear with one or two Cut-Thrus. Like Carol, who sat on her patio using Cut-Thru over and over again, you can repeat these steps until a major emotional or attitudinal shift breaks through—no matter how dark the situation seems.

## Attitude Shifts

Our attitudes form neural circuits in the brain. If we habitually maintain a certain attitude, the brain literally rewires itself to facilitate that attitude. In other words, the brain grows accustomed to certain attitudes.

Many of the things you think of as "you" are nothing more than the neural pathways you've created by repeatedly assuming certain attitudes. We might say that *states*, when reinforced, produce *traits*. Who you are, what you like, and how you respond have been built into your brain by your habits. In a sense, these traits are "you" because they're now hardwired into your brain; but they didn't have to be, and they don't have to stay that way.

That's why, when you *do* get to the deep heart, one of the most beneficial things you can sincerely ask for is the power to make an attitude shift (if one is needed). This takes courage, because mature attitude shifts sometimes move us in a direction that the mind doesn't want to go. The mind has been programmed into certain attitudes and constructs that it doesn't want to release, even if you intuitively know that they're not good for you. And the mind, not knowing what lies ahead if it goes the heart's way, is afraid of risk. So it's sometimes hard to learn to follow the heart.

Sometimes the solutions to problems are right in front of us, but they're blocked from view by negative feelings or old attitudes. Not all problems require a shift in attitude if we're going to reach a solution, but the main ones do—the problems that undermine us. In those cases, attitude shifts often clear the way for tangible solutions. But if we're unwilling to pay the price of making an attitude shift, we block out potential solutions and clarity.

Sometimes people resist shifting out of certain attitudes because they want to reserve the mind's right to pout. People like to pout when they're upset or feel justified in their thwarted point of view. Yet often solutions and insights are blocked because the mind chooses to pout rather than let go of principle. Pouting crystallizes attitudes, thereby keeping you from shifting into what's best for yourself and others.

CUT-THRU allows you to move into new feelings and attitudes, showing you a bigger picture that gets beyond pouting and holding on to inefficient emotions and insecurities. Just keep honoring your commitment to take the significance out and decrease the emotional drain.

## Practicing CUT-THRU

Take some time to study and experiment with the six CUT-THRU steps. As you practice, you'll find that the steps begin to flow easily from one to another. The process will get simpler in a very short time. As we mentioned, you can develop buzzwords or use the highlighted key words to trigger your memory of each step.

The easiest way to learn the steps is to practice each one as you read it. At first, practice with your eyes closed if that's comfortable for you. As you become familiar with the internal process, you'll be able to do it quickly with your eyes open. After awhile, the steps will become automatic and you'll be able to do them anywhere—in the shower, driving in the car, sitting in a meeting.

You can also try doing CUT-THRU to music. Use music that you feel connects you with the heart—something that's not too stimulating, but not too soft and gentle either. Instrumental music that falls somewhere between lively and sleepy works best. Accompanied by the right music, the CUT-THRU technique can become even more powerful. Try experimenting with different music until you find the right style or selection that works for you. The effectiveness of the technique, however, doesn't in any way depend upon music. Learning and applying the technique with sincerity is the most beneficial way to gain from CUT-THRU, whether or not you enhance it musically. (See Chapter 10 for more on the use of music in inner work.)

To become comfortable with the CUT-THRU technique, practice it with the help of the CUT-THRU worksheet on page 198. You can tackle any of the recurring deficit emotions or overcares that you identified in yourself while reading Chapters 7 and 8. You can also try cutting through some of the most common draining emotions listed below. CUT-THRU can help you understand how these emotions operate and facilitate their release.

| | | |
|---|---|---|
| tension | edginess | pain |
| rage | guilt | feeling overwhelmed |
| apathy | hurt | sadness |
| low energy/fatigue | grief | resentment |
| worry | anger | anxiety |
| self-blame | depression | fear |

## Time Pressure

At our trainings, the majority of people tell us that the mood they have the most trouble with is *feeling overwhelmed*. That feeling can lead to edginess, angst, and low-energy fatigue. Doctors tell us that up to 30 percent of their new-patient visits are for unusual or low-energy fatigue, a symptom accompanied more often than not by a chronic sense of being overwhelmed. The most common cause of these feelings is *time pressure*.

But can we really use the CUT-THRU technique to reduce the pressure of time constraints? After all, time pressures seem so external, so out of our control. Our workload, our kids, our volunteer commitments, our household chores—all these make unrelenting demands on our time.

# CUT-THRU Worksheet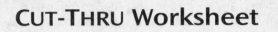

**Here are the six steps of the CUT-THRU technique:**

Step 1—Be Aware of how you Feel about the issue at hand.

Step 2—Focus in the Heart and Solar Plexus—Breathe love and appreciation through this area for 10 seconds or more to help anchor your attention there.

Step 3—Assume Objectivity about the feeling or issue—as if it were someone else's problem.

Step 4—Rest in Neutral—in your Rational, Mature Heart

Step 5—Soak and Relax any disturbed or perplexing feelings in the compassion of the heart—Dissolving the Significance a little at a time. (No time limit.) Take your time doing this step. Remember it's not the problem that causes energy drain as much as the significance you assign to the problem.

Step 6—After Extracting as much Significance as you can, from your Deep Heart sincerely Ask for appropriate guidance or insight. If you don't get an answer: Find something to Appreciate for awhile. Appreciation of anything often facilitates intuitive clarity on issues you were working on.

**Emotional Issue** _____

_____

**Emotional Reactions** _____

_____

_____

_____

_____

### CUT-THRU

**CUT-THRU Response** _____

_____

_____

_____

_____

Well, think of it this way. When we're under pressure and racing against time, it's not just that we feel overwhelmed; we get edgy. And when we're edgy, we often say or do things we wish we hadn't. Then we have to go back and pick up the pieces. That's time lost.

By cutting through feelings of pressure and edginess as soon as you notice them, you come back into emotional balance, and that creates a *time shift*. In other words, you save time because you don't have to go through all the inefficient consequences of moodiness. You can manage yourself *within a time span*—right in the moment—by using CUT-THRU.

In our earlier example of getting up in the morning on the wrong side of the bed, if you'd used CUT-THRU right after you noticed the effects of the first cross words with your spouse, you would have diverted all the negative mental and emotional outplay of that mood at the office (and perhaps again in the evening with your spouse). That's a great deal of time (and energy) saved. Think of how you could have used that time differently.

Using CUT-THRU to shift your emotions and align them with the heart at any time causes a time shift; it stops a chain reaction that results in time waste. You shift into a new time and energy zone of effectiveness. If you forget to CUT-THRU immediately, don't think that you've totally missed the opportunity. Cutting through at *any* moment prevents the loss of time and energy. As you practice the technique repeatedly, the steps will pop up in memory at earlier stages in the chain reaction.

Let's look at a couple of examples. When you're under time pressure and are striving to accomplish certain tasks by a certain time, at least do Step 4: take some of the significance out of the situation instead of floundering in disturbed emotions or letting them affect you like a low-grade fever. And when you're in a meeting and someone says something that disturbs you, go to Step 5: try assigning the disturbed feeling to the heart to soak for the rest of the meeting. Each time you *actualize* an effort of practice, you stop some of the energy drain and create a time shift. As you stack up time shifts, you build new emotional buoyancy and stamina.

About two years ago, I (Howard) had an interesting opportunity to apply CUT-THRU. Using that technique, I was able to create a time shift out of what could have been a tremendous time and energy loss.

One of our employees who was going through a difficult time constantly blamed and judged the people and practices around him. This tendency not only made him miserable, but it started affecting his job and his relationships with his co-workers.

After a meeting at which he was unusually upset, I paused and got beyond my feelings of overcare. Then I entered into a frank discussion with him about his attitude, trying to help him break through. Reacting negatively—and strongly—he told me how much he resented my perspective.

A few days later, he asked me to step outside the building for a moment. He then proceeded to download his wrath, accusing me of having no compassion or sensitivity and blaming me for playing a major role in all of his problems. As his rage increased, he began to challenge me physically. Managing to get to neutral, I held my ground and did the best I could to let him vent his anger.

Once he was through, I went to my office and closed the door. Although I made every effort to stay balanced, I was somewhat shaken. Emotionally charged thoughts about this incident kept churning inside me.

When I realized what was happening, I made a decision to stop everything and sincerely apply CUT-THRU. I went through the steps several times, gaining new perspectives as I went, taking the significance out and soaking my fragile emotions in the heart.

From my rational, mature heart, I was able to see that this colleague was going through a really tough time. Although some employers would have found it appropriate to dismiss him, I knew that he was a dedicated worker with a deep heart. I decided to keep working toward a solution.

After practicing CUT-THRU for awhile that day, I did find some release. As day went into night, though, I still felt a bit unstable, so I kept soaking the remnants of my disturbance to try to bring my emotions back into coherence. It worked.

I continued to try to talk to him to resolve our differences, and over time we did. He in turn used the HeartMath Solution tools and techniques and got back in touch with his heart. I admired him for that. Today he's a highly valued friend making an important contribution to the company.

The benefits of using CUT-THRU are many. One of the first things you'll notice as you practice this technique is that you build your emotional capabilities and increase your self-motivation. Furthermore, you procrastinate less (because you're in the flow more), you become more sensitive and empathetic with other people (resulting in improved interpersonal communication), and you begin to move through life at the most efficient speed possible—the speed of balance.

In effect, you're building a new grid for relating to yourself and life. You're taking your emotional energy and redirecting it in a productive manner. Try the CUT-THRU technique for a week and make it count. See if it doesn't change some things. Be patient with emotional patterns that take more time to shift.

Even if you need a month to work out an emotional issue that's been reinforced for years, that's still a shortcut to emotional freedom!

## Common Mistakes

Be aware of the two most common mistakes people make when practicing CUT-THRU.

*Mistake 1:* "I understand what you're saying, but my fears and anxieties are just so *different* from other people's." People could fight for days trying to prove whose problems are worse. You'll never know if the technique can work for you unless you give it a try.

*Mistake 2:* "My issue is so deep that there's no way any technique could help. I've tried them all." Thousands have tried to adjust their feeling world through self-help practices, religion, and therapy, and it's often a long process. People believe that they can *think* or *emote* and change an attitude, but changes in the feeling world require heart coherence. They also require consistent and sincere practice, because so many of our perceptions, attitudes, and emotional responses are deeply ingrained in our cellular patterning. [3] This keeps the unsolved mysteries of past emotional experiences locked in our nerve cells and in the circuits they form. Our nerve cells actually retain and store accumulated memories of past and present emotionally charged events. [1]

## Understanding Memory Processing

The experimental study of memory dates back to 1885, when Hermann Ebbinghaus engaged in a series of experiments to study how new information is put into memory storage. He reasoned that to be certain new memories were being formed, he'd need to ensure that a subject wouldn't have any past associations to the material he presented to them.

To force subjects to form new memories, he hit upon the idea of giving subjects verbal material that was so totally unfamiliar to them that they couldn't possibly have any prior association with it. He invented nonsense syllables consisting of two consonants separated by a vowel (e.g., WUX, JEK, ZUP). Ebbinghaus created about 2,300 such syllables, wrote each on a separate slip of paper, and randomly drew from seven to thirty-six slips, creating lists of syllables that were to be serially memorized.

From these simple experiments, he discovered two basic principles. First, he found that memory is "graded"—that is, practice makes perfect. Second, he found that there's a linear relationship between the number of repetitions and the amount of memory retained.

Ebbinghaus also studied forgetting. He found that relearning a list takes less time, with fewer trials, than the original learning. He also discovered that forgetting has at least two components: a rapid initial decline in the first hour, followed by a much more gradual decline that continues for about a month. [4]

This research is the basis for new understandings that the brain uses at least two different processes for memory—processes now commonly called short-term and long-term memory. With short-term memory, the synapse strength— synapses being the place where neurons connect with one another—is modified temporarily, and if we repeat an action or behavior, the connection is further strengthened.

In order for long-term memory of behavioral processes to occur, the nerve cells must do two additional things. First, they must undergo a complicated series of chemical reactions to produce a molecule that turns on particular genes contained in the DNA of the nerve cells. Second, the nerve cells must grow and change structurally. It's in these structural changes in the nerve cells (and in the circuits they form) that repeated attitudes, emotional responses, and behaviors become imprinted. [5]

Memory permits cumulative changes in the brain's perceptual and response systems and accounts for the gradual development of new skills and unconscious emotional response patterns. It allows our past experiences to influence our current behavior, even when we don't consciously recollect those experiences. [6]

Once formed, our unconscious memories affect our in-the-moment perceptions, which in turn affect our body's biochemistry and hormone production. By cutting through emotional energy drains in steps, you can use the power of heart coherence to create and reinforce new cellular structural changes and eliminate feeling-world residues at the cellular level. [3]

## Investigating the Hormonal Impact of CUT-THRU

Emotions and hormones go hand in hand. Our perceptions and moods affect our biochemistry, and our biochemistry in turn influences our moods and behavior. [7]

Why is it that people can recall where they were when President Kennedy was shot, but not, say, where they had lunch the day before yesterday? It's because their emotional reaction to Kennedy's death was significantly stronger than their experience at lunch.

The hormones and neurotransmitters released by a strong emotional stimulus help to embed that emotional memory in our neural circuitry. We remember things in relation to how important they are to us. And we tend to remember strong *negative* emotional states more than *positive* ones.

While strong negative and positive emotional imprints may have been important for survival and evolution in our past, in the next phase of human evolution we'll need more emotional management—and subsequently more control over our hormonal responses—if we hope to improve quality of life.

Does CUT-THRU offer a key to that hormonal control? Institute scientists have long been interested in finding out whether regular practice of the CUT-THRU technique changes levels of two key hormones—DHEA and cortisol.

In the medical community, it's well known that the repeated experience of negative emotions can lead to chronic elevation of cortisol levels, which damages brain cells while decreasing levels of DHEA. As we mentioned in Chapter 3, chronic elevation of cortisol can also result in increased bone loss, increased fat accumulation (especially around the waist and hips), impaired memory, and the destruction of brain cells. Scientists have also linked low levels of DHEA with a multitude of disorders, including exhaustion, immune disorders, PMS, menopausal difficulties, Alzheimer's disease, obesity, heart disease, and diabetes. There are also significant indications that increased DHEA levels reduce depression, anxiety, memory loss, and cardiovascular disease. Recent clinical tests at the University of California at San Diego show that increased levels of DHEA produce increased feelings of well-being, energy, and vitality. [3, 8–12]

Starting from the hypothesis that the practice of CUT-THRU would alter the level of these hormones in a beneficial direction, the Institute set up a study involving thirty men and women. The test subjects were trained in the CUT-THRU technique and given an audiotape called *Speed of Balance*, which featured music scientifically designed to facilitate emotional balance. [13] Subjects practiced the CUT-THRU technique five days a week while listening to the music and also used CUT-THRU whenever they felt any overcare or distress. Saliva samples were taken to measure DHEA and cortisol levels both before and after one month of practice.

This study was done using an earlier version of CUT-THRU. The basic principle was the same, but the technique was presented in different language. In training people in CUT-THRU over the years, we've gained a wealth of practical, hands-on knowledge, all of which we've incorporated into the more refined version of the technique presented here. We're continuing our research with CUT-THRU, but as you'll see, even the earlier version of the technique had a very dramatic and positive effect on hormonal balance.

After just one month of practice, the subjects showed an average increase of 100 percent in their DHEA levels and an average drop of 23 percent in their cortisol levels (see Figure 9.1). Some subjects tripled and even quadrupled their DHEA levels in one month. [3]

To give you an idea how significant these findings are, the head scientist at the independent lab that analyzed the hormonal results told us that although he'd seen DHEA supplements and other prescriptions raise DHEA in his many years in the field, he'd seen very few that had doubled the level.

Further analysis was performed to test the relationship between self-reported stress and anxiety and cortisol levels. Results showed that the lower the reported anxiety and stress, the lower the cortisol, confirming the reliability of this relationship in the study. Subjects reported no dietary, exercise, or lifestyle changes during that month except for practicing CUT-THRU and listening to *Speed of Balance*. Scientists have suggested that continued regular practice over time could produce even greater results. [3]

This study is especially significant. It confirms that people have the ability to change their hormonal balance—to increase DHEA and to decrease cortisol—without taking drugs or supplements. This points to the fact that our hormonal patterns are responsive to our changing perceptions and emotions. And remember, these impressive results came after just one month's practice of CUT-THRU.

## Investigating the Emotional Impact of CUT-THRU

I n another phase of the study, the Institute's scientists wanted to find out if regular practice of CUT-THRU would significantly reduce negative feelings and stress and significantly increase positive feelings and well-being. As before, participants were instructed to practice the steps of CUT-THRU five days a week (while listening to *Speed of Balance*) and to practice the technique in any situation that caused them overcare, anxiety, or distress. A control group of fifteen people also took the psychological tests but didn't practice CUT-THRU.

Results showed significant increases in positive feelings of caring, warmheartedness (appreciation, kindness, love, forgiveness, acceptance, harmony,

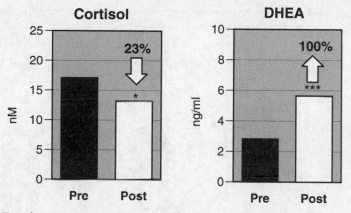

**CUT-THRU's Impact on Hormonal Balance**

FIGURE 9.1. These graphs show levels of the hormones cortisol and DHEA in a group of people before and after they were trained in and had practiced the CUT-THRU technique. After practicing CUT-THRU for one month, subjects had a 23 percent average decrease in cortisol and a 100 percent average increase in DHEA.

© copyright 1998 Institute of HeartMath Research Center

compassion), and vigor, and less substantial increases in contentment and happiness after one month in the group that practiced CUT-THRU. That same group also experienced decreases in anxiety, burnout, depression, guilt, hostility, general overcare, and general stress (see Figure 9.2). In the control group, no significant changes were seen in either positive or negative emotions. [14]

In addition, women in the study kept daily charts of their mood swings during their menstrual cycle for one month prior to learning CUT-THRU and for two months after. The charts revealed marked reductions in mood swings, depression, and fatigue associated with the menstrual period. [14]

These studies illustrate that using CUT-THRU can have a dynamic effect on both our physical and our psychological well-being.

## Taking CUT-THRU Beyond the Lab

These research results are encouraging indeed, but the really good news comes when CUT-THRU makes a significant impact on your own life. And it will—its effects increasing with your practice and commitment.

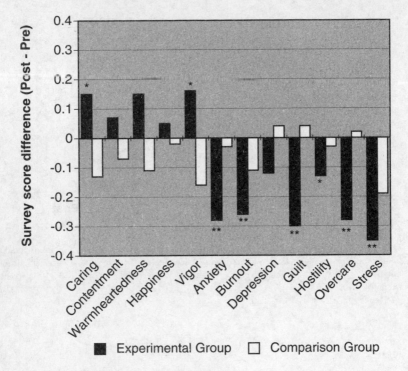

*CUT-THRU's Impact on Emotional Balance*

FIGURE 9.2. After practicing the CUT-THRU technique for one month, study subjects experienced significant reductions in stress, overcare, and negative emotions and increased vigor and positive emotions (black bars). A comparison group that didn't use CUT-THRU showed no significant psychological changes (white bars). *$p$ - .05, **$p$ - .01.

© copyright 1998 Institute of HeartMath Research Center

## Learning to Shift Emotions

Use CUT-THRU whenever you want to make a shift from one emotional state to another. After you become more practiced at this technique, you'll be able to stop emotional drains and shift into more desirable feeling states at will. You'll need a high degree of mastery to shift strong, long-standing emotional patterns at will, but many emotional zones can be cut through quickly.

Suppose you're feeling irritable. Maybe a series of little annoyances have gotten to you. There's nothing big that you can pinpoint, but you're grumpy and on edge all the same. You think about doing a FREEZE-FRAME but decide to follow the steps of CUT-THRU instead, recognizing that your emotional state needs a substantial overhaul. After going through the steps, you find that you've let go of the emotional funk; within a few minutes, you feel a generous sense of appreciation for your experience over the course of the day: nothing major went wrong, and now you've found a flow that allows everything to fall into place. (Not all days are like that, so it's really something to appreciate!) When you cut through a general malaise, a sense of enhanced appreciation rises into your awareness quite naturally.

## Regaining Balance Fast

When your emotions are severely out of balance, it's definitely time to stop whatever you're doing and use CUT-THRU. You might want to do a FREEZE-FRAME first, to try to activate a core heart feeling, and then go on to the CUT-THRU technique. FREEZE-FRAME will help bring your various systems into a more balanced state, thereby making CUT-THRU both easier and more effective. FREEZE-FRAME can get you back into a state of mental clarity and balance quickly, and then CUT-THRU can bring your emotions into coherence with your heart. The two processes are closely related: when, as part of your FREEZE-FRAME, you ask your heart what efficient, stress-minimizing course of action it recommends, you might be told that you need to use CUT-THRU to clear out any leftover distorted emotions.

When we suggest that CUT-THRU should be applied whenever your emotions are severely out of balance, what sorts of occasions are we thinking about? Certainly when you're mad—either during an angry exchange or when the whole thing is over (but you're still fuming and draining energy). And certainly when you're in the grip of strong overcare in one of its many incarnations—worry, for example. As you read this, people all over the world are saying, "This [fill in the blank] is worrying me to death." They may not be kidding.

When you're caught in strong emotions of *any* kind, CUT-THRU can bring you back to balance and poise. And the faster you get back, the more energy you save. You just have to remember to exercise your empowerment and force yourself to slow down to do it. Go through the steps of CUT-THRU until you feel a shift. Remember, you might not instantly feel great. But as you keep cutting through, taking the density and significance out of the feeling or issue, you'll regain your balance. Within a short period of time, your feeling world will make a major shift.

Some problems have no obvious solutions. If you miss a plane to an important meeting and a business deal falls through as a result, you can't change that.

But you *can* take the significance out at the emotional level, regain your balance, and move on. CUT-THRU, sincerely applied, really does help with that. It cuts right through to emotional balance. From head to heart. From chaos to coherence.

## Eliminating the Bigger Blocks

The emotional issues that go way back are usually some of the major blocks that keep us from experiencing greater fulfillment.

Suppose you were deeply hurt in a relationship. The lingering pain you feel won't allow you to express your love, keeping you guarded and insecure. Take these feelings into your heart. Remember, it's not the specific issue that's causing you pain anymore. It's the emotional significance you assigned to it back then and have reinforced all these years. By now the pain is just energy that needs to be transformed so that you can be free to express your love again.

We do understand that getting past emotions that are stored deep in your memory can be hard. But if you really want to move beyond these emotional limitations, set aside time to use CUT-THRU on feelings that you've identified as your major emotional blocks. Once you've targeted them, commit to working through the six CUT-THRU steps on each. As you fulfill that commitment, you'll progressively eliminate your self-defeating patterns. Being vulnerable with yourself will open the heart to bring you the insights you need. In less time than you might think, you'll feel new freedom, release, and comfort as you practice CUT-THRU. Think about how much you might gain from sitting down to do CUT-THRU for thirty minutes or so several days a week for just a month, as the people in the study did, in order to work through an emotional block that's been affecting you for years.

## Generating Your Own Happiness

Because CUT-THRU is a technique that takes you from stressful, taxing emotions to restorative, peaceful ones, it's designed, in a sense, to help you find happiness.

We all want to feel happy, but happiness is a rare commodity. We can't simply *will* it into being, much as we'd like to. The world outside is an equally unreliable source of happiness; if you wait for events and circumstances to make you happy, you'll have a long and often discouraging wait.

The best, most reliable happiness comes from a balanced negotiation between the mind and the heart—a negotiation that takes effort and determination. When emotions get drained through loneliness, jealousy, or fear, there's no emotional fuel left to sustain happiness. Sure, happiness can spring up for a moment, but it doesn't last. Unmanaged emotions suck happiness dry and empty our reserves.

Managing your emotions is an inside job. That's why it's important to learn techniques to make attitude adjustments. You can then direct your emotions more efficiently. Happiness comes through emotions qualified by the heart.

The primary purpose of CUT-THRU is to manage emotions from a place of deep heart intelligence and to quickly arrest emotions that downgrade your happiness. CUT-THRU takes you to the other side of emotional distortion; from that new perspective, you can see a bigger picture and experience greater happiness and inner security.

As your heart gives you insight into what to do differently, it's important to listen and obey. You build your emotional capabilities by actualizing what your heart tells you. Intuitive listening must be followed by intuitive doing. Your happiness depends on it.

## KEY POINTS TO REMEMBER

➤ CUT-THRU facilitates emotional coherence and allows you to transform emotions you don't want into new, regenerative feelings. And it does so without resorting to rationalization or repression.

➤ CUT-THRU isn't an overly simplified self-help technique. It has depth and requires mature reflection and contemplation. Study the steps and make the effort to experiment with the technique.

➤ Use CUT-THRU to shift out of emotions that are draining your energy, regain emotional balance, and eliminate long-standing emotional issues.

➤ The number-one negative mood state that people complain about today is the feeling of being *overwhelmed*. Its basic cause: *time pressure*. By cutting through the feeling of being overwhelmed as soon as you notice it, you come back into emotional balance, and that creates a *time shift*.

➤ Managing your emotions with CUT-THRU requires that you first recognize how you're feeling. Breathing through the heart and solar plexus helps you anchor your emotions. Assuming objectivity leads to emotional maturity.

> Let your heart dissipate inharmonious emotional energy. It's not a particular issue that's causing the problem; it's the emotional energy you've invested in that issue. Taking the significance out of the issue and soaking it in the heart releases stored energy and brings new insights.

> Often old identities keep us feeling stuck. You may not even know what they are. By applying CUT-THRU, you can erase unproductive emotional patterning in your unconscious memory and neural circuitry.

> Emotions and hormones go hand in hand. Our perceptions and moods affect our biochemistry, and our biochemistry in turn influences our moods and behavior.

> The benefits you'll derive from using the CUT-THRU technique are many. One of the first things you'll notice is that you're building your emotional capabilities. In addition, your self-motivation will increase, you'll procrastinate less (because you're in the flow more), you'll become more sensitive and empathetic with other people (resulting in improved interpersonal communication), and you'll begin to move through life at the most efficient speed possible—the speed of balance.

CHAPTER 10

# HEART LOCK-IN

Wouldn't it be wonderful if you could climb into a machine that bombarded you with revitalizing energy? Or if there were a special power place somewhere, high in the mountains or deep in a tropical forest, where you were sure to reach your next level of insight, awareness, and vitality in just a short visit?

Before learning about HeartMath, Deborah, a successful executive with a biotechnology company, used to take trips every few months to the desert or to a Catholic monastic retreat overlooking the ocean in order to gain a new measure of peace, inspiration, and renewed connection with her heart. She loved those quiet, uplifting times—they provided a valuable source of renewal—but, as with most people, Deborah would plunge right back into her busy life and the feeling would fade within a few days.

After Deborah learned and practiced the HEART LOCK-IN technique, she was surprised to find that she was able to gain a sense of renewal and connection with her heart similar to that which she'd found in her retreats. Deborah says, "Nothing satisfies me more than making contact with my heart. I love going away on trips where I can spend time with myself, but that's not always practical. The HEART LOCK-IN is something I can do every day to bring me to that place of balance and heart resonance in fifteen minutes and sustain that feeling into my day. I no longer feel the same need to get away from it all and retreat. I can now find that retreat in my own heart wherever I am."

When you get deeply in touch with your heart, it's like discovering your own internal tropical forest, ocean, or mountain peak waiting to refresh you. We all know it's there. It's the place inside of us that we hope to find when we take a vacation or a walk in nature.

Once you begin to regularly use the FREEZE-FRAME and CUT-THRU techniques found in the previous chapters, you'll experience significant relief from the everyday stresses of your life. After you've eliminated some of the blocks that have dogged your path, the world will start to look better. You'll naturally be more appreciative, more forgiving, and less judgmental. Problems won't seem so insurmountable. Your heart intelligence will be more active and readily available. You'll see a bigger picture, and that's what brings hope.

With FREEZE-FRAME improving the communication between your heart and brain, your mental acuity will increase. Your practice of CUT-THRU will be bringing your emotions back into balance and giving you access to new intuitive intelligence by eliminating old emotional blocks. Together, these two tools will noticeably reduce your energy deficits and help you build reliable energy assets.

Although it may not have been your original intention, you'll also like yourself more. That means that relationships will improve. The more your core heart values come into play, the more you'll wonder, "What else is there? How else can I learn and develop?" Your new loving, openhearted perspective will cause you to ask what other ways you can help others and continue to grow.

HEART LOCK-IN is the technique to use to go deeper in the heart to explore the richer textures and expanded awareness that reside there. HEART LOCK-INS are used not necessarily to solve a specific problem but rather to give you a pleasurable, regenerative experience and greater overall access to the intuitive intelligence of the heart. In this regard, HEART LOCK-IN is different from FREEZE-FRAME or CUT-THRU. While these latter techniques can be used for more than problem-solving—they're useful for increasing coherence to enhance creativity and awareness about any subject matter, for example—more often we use them when we need to find a solution or shift from a less-than-optimal state of mind to one that's more coherent and effective. HEART LOCK-IN, on the other hand, is used for deeper relaxation, regeneration, and awareness, and to enhance the effectiveness of the other HeartMath Solution tools and techniques.

If you're going to establish an important relationship with this dawning new intelligence within you, you have to devote time to developing that bond. As in any other relationship, you have to address problems that interfere with your communication and clear up issues that get in the way. But the most important thing is to spend time together.

The HEART LOCK-IN technique gives you a five- to fifteen-minute dose of quality time with your heart. Because it can set the tone for the whole day, it's good to practice first thing in the morning. That way you start off in the right direction before the chaos of the day kicks in.

FREEZE-FRAME and CUT-THRU do wonders for clearing away incoherence—they're like pulling weeds in a garden—while HEART LOCK-IN nourishes the soil. This technique has been designed to help you cultivate an even more enriched relationship with your heart. It's a potent technique that you can use any time you want to deepen the most important connection in your life. [1]

## Your Deepest Heart

The HEART LOCK-IN technique is designed to help you amplify the power of your heart and the power of your love. As you cultivate the wonderful field of the heart within you, you regenerate your life—physically, mentally, emotionally, and spiritually. Your life begins to respond to a new energy.

"It's hard to describe," one seminar participant said, "but the emotions I feel now seem to be richer, more textured. There's a casual sense of peace. I'm more relaxed than I've been in years, but at the same time, I feel more acutely aware of my environment."

In the HEART LOCK-IN technique, you focus your energies in the area of your heart for five to fifteen minutes (or longer, if you like). It's very similar to Step 2 of FREEZE-FRAME, except that here your focus is more gentle. As you sustain your attention in the heart for a longer period of time, you reap more benefits and create a more enduring connection with the heart.

Quieting the mind and sustaining a solid connection with the heart—*locking in* to its power—adds buoyancy and regenerative energy to your entire system. As you lock in your coherent heart rhythms to sustain the entrainment state we talked about before, you begin to refine the energy that emanates from the heart, retraining and reprogramming your nervous system and reorganizing your cells, organs, and electrical system. With practice, entrainment becomes your natural state. Why not try it right now?

## Practicing HEART LOCK-IN

Here's how you do it:

1. Find a quiet place, close your eyes, and try to relax.
2. Shift your attention away from the mind or head and focus your attention in the heart area. Pretend that you're breathing slowly through the heart for ten or fifteen seconds.

3. Remember the feeling of love or care you have for someone whom it's easy for you to love. Alternatively, focus on a feeling of appreciation for someone or something positive in your life. Try to stay with that feeling for a time from five to fifteen minutes.

4. Gently send that feeling of love, care, or appreciation to yourself or others.

5. As head thoughts come in, bring your focus gently back to the area around the heart. If the energy feels too intense or feels blocked, try to feel a softness in the heart and relax.

6. After you've finished, if you can, write down any intuitive feelings or thoughts that are accompanied by a sense of inner knowingness or peace to help you remember to act on them.

Unlike FREEZE-FRAME, a HEART LOCK-IN isn't about asking a specific question or looking for answers, as we noted earlier. Instead, you focus on finding *core heart feelings* such as sincere appreciation, true care, and compassion or love, and maintaining these states. Intuitive answers will often come anyway, however. You consult your heart in LOCK-INS, but you let answers find you instead of looking for them.

Sending out core heart feelings—radiating them throughout your body and cells or radiating them to other people or issues—helps you lock into the feeling state (and thus the coherence state) longer. With a little practice, you'll be able to slow down the mind and find your way more quickly to your core heart feelings. It's an "easy does it" process, not something you force or will yourself into.

Remember those holographic pictures, or stereograms, that were popular a few years ago? When you first looked at them, all you could see was a mass of colorful dots. Then, as you relaxed and shifted your vision slightly, a magnificent, detailed picture took shape among the dots. The key to getting the picture to emerge was to relax and not try too hard to see it. Likewise, one key to maximizing your HEART LOCK-IN experience is to relax and not try too hard.

Your ability to relax into a HEART LOCK-IN will allow you to find the appropriate feelings and break through into new experiences, insights, and perceptions. Your skill at achieving this goal will develop naturally in accordance with your sincere heart efforts.

But obviously you can't reap the rewards without cultivating the practice. The first step is to make the time to do a HEART LOCK-IN every day. We're talking about only five to fifteen minutes, remember. In return, you'll build up your energy reserves, deepen intuition, and stay longer in an intuitive flow.

Intuition can manifest in very practical ways. Though elements of intuition are mysterious, HEART LOCK-IN isn't an inherently mystical experience; both the process and the results are tangible, offering many commonsense advantages. Jennifer Weil, a middle school teacher, tells how the technique helped ensure that her English honors students would be able to demonstrate their knowledge on an important exam.

Jennifer's twenty high school students were assembled on a hot afternoon to take the English placement exam for honors English. They had only an hour to complete the essay they'd been assigned, but Jennifer took more than five of those precious minutes to do a HEART LOCK-IN with them.

"During the hour," Jennifer said, "I watched as several students closed their eyes again, placed their hands on their hearts for a moment, then continued their essays. Every student finished calmly and easily, and all but one was accepted into the honors program on the basis of their work that afternoon."

## Sending Core Heart Feelings

The practice of radiating core heart feelings such as love, care, and appreciation in HEART LOCK-INS has many beneficial effects. HEART LOCK-INS help you sustain the entrainment state that provides a foundation for healing in the body and in relationships. Your heart rhythms come into coherence for a longer period of time, which helps increase coherence within all the body's systems—mental, emotional, spiritual, electrical, and cellular. Sustaining coherence creates alignment with your deeper, mature heart, which brings you into warm contact with your personal source of spirit.

When people send out their core heart feelings, they often report that they can actually feel the heart energy—as a warmth around the heart; as a liquid feeling, as if it were a pool or river of love, care, or appreciation; as circles of energy expanding from the heart; or as a tingling in the cells.

As people continue to radiate core heart feelings to others or to life, they sense the love, care, or appreciation as a tangible energy connecting them to people and nature. That connection feels wonderful—soothing to the emotions, mind, and body.

Moreover, when people send love and care to someone with whom they're having problems, the relationship often improves. Whether this is due to the sender's making an attitude shift or to the receiver's making a thought or feeling shift is a question that perhaps quantum physics may someday be able to explain. Whatever the reason, though, the more love and care you send out toward a person (or issue), the more you come into alignment both with your spirit and with that person, and the more your intuition comes on-line.

After Carolyn had been in her new job for eight months, she found out that she was going to have to move out of town in the near future for personal reasons. When she told Linda, the director who was still training her, their connection became very strained. Carolyn felt guilty but didn't know what she could do about it.

Still feeling bad several days later, she remembered to do a HEART LOCK-IN. As she radiated love and care to Linda, she hoped to find a deeper connection between them. During the LOCK-IN, she got the idea of writing Linda a letter expressing her feelings.

What happened next surprised her. "The very next day," Carolyn said, "before I had a chance to write the letter, Linda dropped by my office and started a warm conversation. We discovered that we'd had some similar experiences in our lives, and Linda told me she wished me well when I moved to Boston."

"That was my cue. I apologized for putting her through this situation, and she sincerely thanked me. It gave me the chance to tell her how much I appreciated her from my heart. All the things I was going to say in my letter flowed out."

Because Carolyn had enhanced her core heart feelings in the HEART LOCK-IN, she was ready to recognize and make use of the opportunity to sincerely connect with Linda on the spot. Carolyn said that she'd never talked to a co-worker at that level before, and both women benefited from the experience.

## Spirituality and Health

Our values and beliefs can determine our successes and failures in life. But can they determine our health?

Numerous studies are showing correlations between belief, personal values, and healing, and the medical community is starting to acknowledge that medicine's reluctance to tackle "spiritual" issues may hamper public health.

C. Everett Koop, who was the surgeon general of the United States in the 1980s, says that the attitude of the medical community toward spirituality has come full circle. When he first went into medicine sixty years ago, doctors were taught to use their patients' beliefs to help them heal. By the late 1950s and 60s, faith and spirituality became absolutely taboo. Now mind/body medicine is so much in the public eye that the medical community is welcoming back the spirituality, faith, and prayer principles once again. [2]

The question of just what spirituality is is part of the problem. People can be spiritual but not religious, or religious with little feeling for their own spirituality. Many people agree that spirituality includes having a sense of purpose in life, a deep personal value system, and a feeling of deep connectedness with oneself, other people, and "spirit"—some form of higher power or intelligence. If health is viewed as wholeness, then we must incorporate spirit along with the body, mind, and emotions for a whole and healthy self.

Famous for researching and developing noninvasive methods of treating heart disease, Dr. Dean Ornish found that heart disease could be relieved and in some cases reversed when patients made significant changes in diet and exercise and used meditation and support groups to help relieve stress. After years of teaching and writing books on his methods, Ornish concluded in his latest book, *Love and Survival*, that it was the love that heart patients felt through intimately opening their hearts in support groups that had the greatest stress relief and healing benefit. [3]

Many of the most popular books on the bestseller list in the nineties have addressed spirituality and the relationship between spirit, love, mind, and body. Polls show that four out of five Americans believe spirituality is related to health. [4] Dr. Herbert Benson, in his book *Timeless Healing*, describes how he became convinced from his medical practice that our bodies are genetically hardwired to benefit from our rich inner core—our beliefs, values, thoughts, and feelings, and how he attempted to research these seemingly intangible aspects of being human. [5]

Benson developed a technique called "the relaxation response" to help people calm themselves and improve their health. In this technique, patients close their eyes and repeat a one- or few-word relaxation statement of their choice—perhaps one that reflects their values, whether a prayer or even the simple word "one"—to help them calm down. Benson found that 25 percent of those he questioned felt "more spiritual" as a result. They described the experience as the presence of an energy, a force, a power beyond themselves, and they reported that the presence felt close to them.

After practicing medicine for many years, Dr. Larry Dossey was stunned to discover scientific evidence for the healing power of prayer. Intrigued, he embarked on ten years of research into the relationship between prayer and healing.

In his book *Healing Words*, Dossey examines which methods of prayer show the greatest potential for healing. While he found that all types of prayer help, studies have shown that prayers sent without a specific outcome in mind, "letting the universe do the work," yield scientific results that are twice as great. [6]

Dossey's book talks about the importance of surrendering the mind and choosing a method of prayer that intuitively feels best. He sums up his years of research in these words: "As we recognize the empirical evidence for prayer's power . . . we will find ourselves praying more prayers of gratitude and fewer prayers of supplication . . . realizing the world, at heart, is more glorious, benevolent, and friendlier than we have recently supposed."

## Balance—A Personal Choice

Before developing the HEART LOCK-IN technique, I (Doc) practiced prayer and meditation at least five hours a day, five days a week for years. This regular practice, along with my research into various techniques, led me to new discoveries—discoveries that eventually evolved into the HeartMath Solution. I wasn't trying, in my research and practice, to reinvent the wheel on either prayer or meditation; rather, I was trying to *ground* them, to bring sky to street.

In the South, where I grew up, Baptist revivals and prayer meetings were a way of life. From an early age, I used prayer to find guidance and inspiration. Later, when I decided to research prayer's effects, I practiced many forms of prayer and its close relative, meditation. I realized that people have their own interpretation of what *prayer* and *meditation* mean, yet I encountered some common elements.

It troubled me that even in southern culture, where prayer was common, most people had trouble bringing insights gained from prayer or meditation into everyday life. I began to realize that those who did it most successfully were those who had the best emotional management and balance in their lives. The trouble wasn't with prayer; it was with the emotional state of the people who practiced it. So I began to look for ways to help.

I foresaw that stress would be increasing dramatically in society and realized that millions of people didn't know about—and probably wouldn't practice— formal meditation techniques. But they were going to need something very practical to reduce their mental and emotional stress and give them a stronger inner sense of well-being.

The HeartMath Solution was created to provide new ways to assist people through these challenges. I particularly designed HEART LOCK-IN to help people stay balanced and grounded, knowing that this would allow them to actualize more heart in their daily lives. My motive has always been to help people live more in the way of love and love each other more—whatever their beliefs, religion, or spiritual practices might be.

I like to call HEART LOCK-IN a "beneficial facilitator." It's not competitive, and it doesn't detract from anyone's beliefs or approach to going within. I knew, as I developed this technique, that many existing techniques were very helpful. I'd gotten a lot of personal benefit from my earlier practice in a wide range of meditation techniques and other inner work.

HEART LOCK-IN enriched rather than replaced the various practices and techniques I used. I found that it enhanced my ability to pray sincerely and to put my insights into action. Once I'd refined HEART LOCK-IN within myself, I found that it gave me the essence of what I'd been getting out of my other practices. By putting HEART LOCK-IN at the center of my inner work and giving up some of the other practices, I gained more time to keep up with my research and work intensities. Most important, that approach helped me to keep my life in balance.

Balance is a key factor in achieving our goals in any area of life—in relationships, diet, exercise, sleep, reading, prayer, meditation, and so on. But what's balanced for one person may be imbalanced for another, and what's balanced for someone today may be different from what it was five years ago and what it will be next year. Many of the staff at HeartMath have changed their diet or exercise programs many times over the years. Some of us were vegetarians for ten or fifteen years, for example, but now find it more appropriate to eat a balanced diet of meat, vegetables, and grains. At this point in our lives this wider program suits us, while other programs were proper before.

Practical living means knowing what's balanced for you as an individual. All people are different. By listening to your heart, you can find your own balance. HEART LOCK-INS provide an excellent way to consult your heart to find balance in any area of your life, including diet, exercise, inner-work techniques, and how much to work and how much to play.

Remember, the purpose of doing HEART LOCK-INS is to help you strengthen the communication link between your heart and brain and sustain entrainment and coherence for longer periods. Doing LOCK-INS regularly builds your heart power to keep your nervous, immune, and hormonal systems in balance. Doing LOCK-INS increases the amount of time your heart is on-line, making it easier to activate core heart feelings and use techniques such as FREEZE-FRAME or CUT-THRU (or other practices you enjoy).

## Locking in with Music

We know that music can shift our feelings and attitudes. Have you ever been at a party with fast-paced dance music playing in the background when somebody suddenly decided to put on an old blues album? The exciting, nervous rhythm in the room is abruptly replaced by a slow, moody rhythm. Someone with a mournful, ragged voice begins to sing. What happens in the room? The dance steps change to accommodate the new music, but the *feeling* all around you changes too.

Music can excite you, relax you, make you happy or nostalgic. It can even evoke a dramatic story. Think about a movie soundtrack, for example. At Heart-Math, we use music as an "atmospheric conditioner," creating an environment that makes it easier to feel the heart. [7–9]

Doing a HEART LOCK-IN with music is one of the best ways to increase the effectiveness of your experience. Find music that feels right for you. As in doing CUT-THRU with music, we suggest using instrumental music that falls somewhere between stimulating and peaceful. Use music that you feel helps open your heart and promote internal balance but doesn't space you out or make you drowsy. Remember, HEART LOCK-INS are designed to give you a relaxed *but highly aware* experience.

## HEART LOCK-INS and Your Body

HEART LOCK-INS are like vitamins for your immune system. One of the Institute's research studies focused on changes in an immune antibody known as secretory IgA as subjects did HEART LOCK-INS with and without music. As we said in Chapter 8, secretory IgA is the body's first line of defense against invading pathogens. Found throughout the mucous linings of the body, it's an important measurement of immune system health. [10]

In the first phase of this experiment, study participants' IgA levels were measured before and after doing a fifteen-minute HEART LOCK-IN while attempting to feel sincere appreciation. After the HEART LOCK-IN, average IgA levels in the group increased by 50 percent, a significant increase in this important immune system marker. A second phase of the experiment was conducted several days later. This time, participants were instructed to do a fifteen-minute HEART LOCK-IN attempting to feel appreciation while listening to the music *Heart Zones*, which was scientifically designed to facilitate internal coherence. [11] Amazingly, the group showed a 141 percent increase in IgA levels. [7] (See Figure 10.1.)

During both phases of the experiment, researchers monitored the autonomic nervous system of each participant. An increase in total autonomic activity was observed in all of the subjects. The study demonstrated that the HEART LOCK-IN technique produced an immuno-enhancing effect mediated by increased autonomic activity, and the immuno-enhancing effect was increased when subjects practiced the technique while listening to *Heart Zones*.

Whether you do HEART LOCK-INS with or without music, this technique is an important part of the HeartMath Solution. Taking that five to fifteen minutes as often as you can to lock in to deeper heart feelings is a sincere act of self-care. With the right music, HEART LOCK-INS may become your favorite technique, but don't feel that you need music to make it work for you. The heart stands on its own.

## Going Deep and Wide

A funny thing we've noticed is that when people practice HEART LOCK-INS, they often tend to want to let the expansive feeling go into the head. So many techniques—creative visualization and some forms of meditation, for example—teach people to create a feeling of expanded consciousness in the head. This can be stimulating, but it can also leave you feeling ungrounded. The purpose of a HEART LOCK-IN is to stay focused in the heart, not the head, so you stay balanced and grounded.

Going to the head can be a habit that's hard to break. After all, when you shut your eyes and start to tune out day-to-day thoughts, you may feel a sense of detachment and an enjoyable widening of the mind. This expanded sense can produce grand thoughts and creative ideas. One idea just leads to another.

Raoul has been a devoted meditator for years. He developed his own routine around meditation and by now can experience deep relaxation after a few minutes. The trouble is that if the phone rings or somebody knocks on his door, he

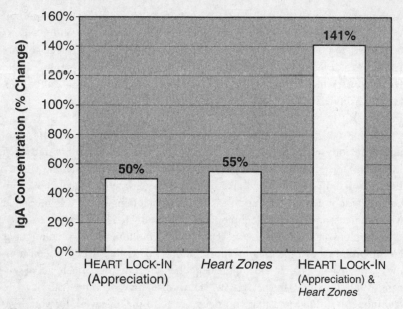

*Effects of HEART LOCK-IN on the Immune System*

FIGURE 10.1. This graph illustrates average changes in the immune antibody secretory IgA in a group of people after doing a HEART LOCK-IN; after listening to *Heart Zones,* music scientifically designed to facilitate mental and emotional balance; and after doing a HEART LOCK-IN facilitated with the *Heart Zones* music. All three conditions significantly increased IgA levels, but the greatest immuno-enhancement was achieved when the *Heart Zones* music was used in conjunction with the HEART LOCK-IN technique.

© copyright 1998 Institute of HeartMath Research Center

has a hard time getting back from what he's been experiencing in the inner world. He finds it very jarring to try to reorient himself to the real world and deal with the interruption, because he's not grounded.

The goal of HEART LOCK-IN is to try to go deep in the heart first. From there you can experience an expanded awareness while staying poised and balanced. If something interrupts you, you may require a little adjustment, certainly; but since you're not spaced out, you can be flexible and adjust fast—taking care of whatever needs to be done and coming back to your LOCK-IN afterwards. The idea is to be present, grounded, and expanded all at the same time.

If you're like most people when you're doing a HEART LOCK-IN, you'll have wide, inspiring thoughts and ideas. This can be enjoyable, entertaining, and at times illuminating. There's nothing wrong with that, but try not to get lost in such thoughts. The trick is to acknowledge the thoughts or images when they arise, enjoy them for a moment, then gently return your attention to the core feelings of the heart. You don't want to get caught up in *concepts* about the heart; you want to stay in the *feeling* qualities of the heart. This helps to keep the mind and heart in balance.

By staying deep and managing wide, you energize your mental, emotional, and physical systems more than if you float off into the mind. In surrendering the mind to the heart, you won't be giving up anything. Going deep won't take the fun out of HEART LOCK-INS. All of your plans, creative ideas, and insights will still be there when you get through. After your LOCK-IN is over, you'll find that you have a connection to the heart that you can carry forward into the rest of your day. You'll be "present" with more of your faculties and be able to in-creasingly sustain a state of flow in your activities.

## You and Yourself

D on't underestimate the depth of what goes on when you do a HEART LOCK-IN. It develops the most important relationship of all—the rela-tionship between you and yourself. Become your own scientist and experiment with it.

Try to do a fifteen-minute HEART LOCK-IN three to five times a week. If you can find the right music, listen to it when doing these LOCK-INS. If you need to be calm for a test (as in the example of the middle school students), need to be prepared for a potentially contentious meeting, or need a boost of energy during the day and can get away for a few minutes, do a five-minute HEART LOCK-IN.

Connect with your heart deeply and send love and care to any area of your life or to your body—either generally or to a specific organ or system. See if things don't work out better.

Down the road, as you keep making the shift from head to heart, you'll in-creasingly feel as if you're living in the heart all the time. You'll take care of busi-ness and all your activities and relationships from a grounded yet openhearted state. Your connection to the heart will always be there, in varying degrees, from dawn to dusk. In fact, *it already is.* Using the HEART LOCK-IN technique is about learning how to spend more time in that place of connection. After a certain point, though, it begins to feel as if that connected state is just who you are. When you've reached that point, HEART LOCK-INS won't feel like trying to get somewhere. They'll be an easy way to go to where you already are.

It's just common sense to go for that feeling of knowingness inside. Not only does it bring benefits to every area of your life, but it feels great as well. But here's the secret: no one else is going to do it for you. No one else is going to give you fulfillment on a silver platter. Your security lies within you, just waiting for you to find it.

## KEY POINTS TO REMEMBER

➤ The HEART LOCK-IN technique helps you discover that you have your own internal source of regeneration.

➤ Quieting the mind and sustaining a solid connection with the heart— *locking in* to its power—adds buoyancy and regenerative energy to your entire system.

➤ The more your core heart feelings come into play, the more you realize how much can be gained from a loving, openhearted perspective.

➤ The practice of radiating core heart feelings such as love, care, and appreciation in HEART LOCK-INS has many beneficial effects. HEART LOCK-INS help you enter and maintain the entrainment state, which provides a foundation for healing in the body and in relationships.

➤ Studies show that the HEART LOCK-IN technique produces an immuno-enhancing effect mediated by increased autonomic activity, and the immuno-enhancing effect is increased when subjects practice the technique while listening to the music *Heart Zones*.

➤ HEART LOCK-INS help to increase coherence within all the body's systems—spiritual, mental, emotional, electrical, and cellular. Coherence brings you into entrainment and alignment with your deeper, mature heart.

PART 4

# Social Heart Intelligence

Parts I through III of *The HeartMath Solution* have given you tools and techniques to help you follow your heart. Experience tells us that those who apply these tools and techniques consistently notice a tremendous improvement in many aspects of their personal lives. Application of the HeartMath Solution goes beyond the personal benefits, however.

Throughout this book we've presented science, case studies, personal experiences, and anecdotes illustrating the power of applied heart intelligence. In Part IV we'll take these applications further.

First, we'll show how heart intelligence can be (and already is being) applied to produce significant positive changes in our families, businesses, communities, and society. We'll start with improvements in families and educational systems. Some of the most hopeful and dramatic results have come when parents and educators have used the HeartMath Solution with children.

Most of us work in a company or organization. One of the primary applications of the HeartMath Solution has been to enhance productivity and increase job satisfaction in the workplace. We'll present information showing the effects of applying the tools and techniques in organizational settings.

Finally, we'll discuss what the emergence of heart intelligence means for society and the world as a whole. Rapid change and new challenges are impacting everyone in all nations. We'll offer our view of the current state of our global society and suggest ways to apply the HeartMath Solution to meet challenges, manage change, and make a valuable contribution to a world in need of new intelligence and more heart.

In Part IV you will:

➤ See how the HeartMath Solution tools and techniques can be used with children.

➤ Realize the effectiveness of applying heart intelligence in organizations and in community improvement efforts.

➤ Better understand our current era of high-speed transformation and perceive how to remain balanced in the midst of change.

# CHAPTER 11

# Families, Children, and the Heart

Imagine what it would be like if we could give our families and communities a feeling of safety and security, of hope and optimism for the future. What if those around us were able to have significantly greater balance and control in their lives—even in the midst of change? In the previous chapters, we've learned how to use FREEZE-FRAME, the heart power tools, CUT-THRU, and HEART LOCK-IN to engage our heart intelligence and create a more coherent state within ourselves. As we radiate our heart coherence to people and issues around us, we'll find that relationships become smoother and solutions to problematic issues come easier. The HeartMath Solution will change the way we address our family, workplace, and societal problems.

## Family Values

Family is the primary social unit in which we can develop the qualities of the heart. A true family grows and moves through life together, inseparable in the heart. Whether a biological family or an extended family of people attracted to each other based on heart resonance and mutual support, the word "family" implies warmth and a place where the core feelings of the heart can be nurtured.

Family values represent the core values and guidelines that parents and family members hold in high regard for the well-being of the family. Sincere family feelings are core heart feelings; they're the basis for true family values. While we have differences, we remain "family" by virtue of our heart connection. Family provides necessary security and support and acts as a buffer against external problems. A family made up of secure people generates a magnetic power that can get things done. They're the hope for real security in a stressful world.

Unfortunately, many families today aren't the secure haven we wish they were. Many people believe that the modern family is dangerously near extinction because of increased family instability and a decline in family values. Family structures have changed dramatically since the 1970s. [1] Families have become smaller and more fractured. More are led by one parent or a grandparent or a stepparent.

Family values remain important to most parents, according to a 1992 Massachusetts Mutual Life Insurance Company survey of 1,050 American adults. In a report titled "Communicating Family Values," Massachusetts Mutual notes that Americans define their top three family values as being responsible for one's actions, respecting others for who they are, and providing emotional support for family members. They overwhelmingly believe that family values are taught primarily by parents setting a good example and that the value "providing emotional support" is learned primarily by example. In fact, all that children have to go on is our example. But the "hope of the future" is learning to be just as stressed out and unfulfilled as we are. [2]

The truth is that we can't teach what we don't know. We say we want our children to express core heart values such as respect, loyalty, gratitude, and emotional support, but we seem to expect them to cultivate those qualities on their own. Kids have to be *taught* the value of those things—not by what we say but by how we live.

When parents and children both are emotionally unmanaged, reactive, moody, and anxious, their relationships jam up. Out of reaction, parents demand emotional management from children, yet they haven't learned it themselves. This perpetuates a loop of argumentation, diluting communication and family bonding. The result is insecurity, anxiety, fear projection, and sustained emotional disconnection.

Today's children make up the first generation in the history of the world to receive information directly from the media, without adults to filter it. Parents are wise to be concerned. Without intervention, kids absorb the values they perceive in music, television, and movies. Nine times out of ten, these media put value on what's sizzling, tantalizing, or forbidden—which often means sex, gore, and violence. [3]

As Jeff Goelitz, director of HeartMath's Education and Family Division, points out, "Children's myths come from the media conglomerates instead of their parents and relations. They're not skilled at navigating in this world, yet these kids are on their own trying to make meaning and filter out the good from the bad."

According to Richard Dahl, associate professor of psychiatry and pediatrics at the University of Pittsburgh Medical Center, the average child spends three hours a day in front of the TV set. That's twenty-one hours a week! By contrast, kids spend roughly thirty hours a week in school. Their time with their parents is far less—only eight minutes of "meaningful conversation" with their fathers and eleven minutes with their mothers in an entire week. [4]

With such an incredible lack of quality time spent together, it's no wonder parents come to feel that their influence on their kids is insignificant. Even if they worry, for example, that their teenager is engaging in high-risk behavior such as drinking, smoking, or violence, they aren't sure how to address their concern.

Adolescents are often very skillful at conveying the message that what parents say or do has no influence on their lives, and many parents believe them, feeling powerless and unheard in their efforts to help their kids lead healthy lives. However, a recent study conducted by Michael Resnick, a sociologist at the University of Minnesota, provides strong evidence that parents do make a real difference in the lives of their children, all the way through high school. In the nationwide study, Resnick and his colleagues found that the health and well-being of teenagers depended to a large extent on the feeling of being cared for by their parents. Teenagers who felt loved by their parents did better across the board at avoiding risky behaviors—including early sex, smoking, alcohol and drug abuse, violence, and suicide—regardless of social or economic status. [5]

## The Role of the Heart in Child Development

Feeling loved is more important to and for children than anything else. New research at Harvard University shows that adults who didn't feel loved as children suffer from a much higher rate of disease than those who experienced love. What this means is that love is a requirement, not an option, for a healthy living. [6]

From the moment a child is born, love is as vital to his health and survival as physical nourishment. Although the basic brain structure and neural circuits for managing emotions are laid down well before birth, it's the experiences a baby has in the early years of life that matter most. The emotional environment that a child is exposed to affects the development of his emotional circuitry. [7]

Emotional states are contagious. Smile at a baby and the baby smiles back. Get upset and the baby cries. As we saw earlier, our heart's electromagnetic field extends beyond our bodies and carries information about our emotional states to those around us. When a parent feels genuine love and care, a harmonious, coherent heart rhythm is communicated to her child. When a parent is in a stressful, anxious, or angry state, a disharmonious, incoherent heart rhythm pattern is communicated. As we've shown in previous chapters—for example, in the electricity of touch study discussed in Chapter 8—the electromagnetic communication from our heart radiates outside the body and is felt by others.

Talking or reading to young children can be counterproductive when a parent is anxious, angry, or stressed. If a mother or father is trying to be nice to or read to a child while anxious or emotionally upset, the electromagnetic field produced by the parent's heart is less coherent, and the child's nervous system detects that incoherence.

Parents who express chronic anxiety and/or depression around their children increase the likelihood that their children will suffer from a broad range of mental or emotional problems. One study involving children aged seven to thirteen with parents who were under treatment for a depressive disorder, anxiety disorder, or mixed anxiety/depression disorder found that 36 percent of children with anxious parents had anxiety, 38 percent of children with depressed parents had depression, and 45 percent of children with mixed anxiety/depression parents were eventually diagnosed with that same disorder. [8]

According to the study's lead investigator, Deborah C. Beidel at the Medical University of South Carolina in Charleston, "These findings don't mean that anxiety and other disorders are tied to a specific gene; learning and modeling can be very powerful ways of acquiring behavior."

When a primary caregiver is attuned to the feelings of a child and responds appropriately to the child's emotions, the neural circuits are positively reinforced. However, if a child's emotions are met repeatedly with a response that's indifferent or negating, the neural circuits can become confused. Those weakened connections may not be strong enough to withstand the neural pruning process that occurs around the age of ten or twelve; often they're lost forever. Neurons that haven't made connections or developed circuits are pruned back and dissolved into the surrounding cerebro-spinal fluid to allow other neuronal structures to grow. However, even after parental neglect, there are many examples of children in whom emotional and mental stress has been overcome through the sincere love and care of a foster parent, "big brother," or mentor. [7]

The brain's plasticity offers hope that at any age, emotional circuitry can be "reeducated" by positive reinforcement and by teaching children and adults techniques for emotional self-management.

Children are surprisingly open to emotional self-management techniques (even at an early age) because of their natural emotional resilience. Researchers know that resilience and flexibility start a diminishing curve in adolescence, however. If children aren't taught emotional management skills by the time they become teens, the adolescents of today will become the emotionally unmanaged adults of tomorrow.

Educators like Jeff Goelitz know that the high-speed world these kids are going to graduate into will demand considerable self-reliance and high-speed intuitive intelligence. And the competition will be intense. Mental aptitude is always valuable, of course, but the future will bring a greater need for creative, adaptive skills than ever before. The ability to get along with people and use refined interpersonal and social skills will be essential. This is where heart intelligence comes in.

By using the FREEZE-FRAME technique together, parents and their children can begin to gain new perceptions on family issues such as discipline, responsibilities, communication, and family activities. They can use CUT-THRU to help find solutions and release from highly charged emotional episodes. And they can use HEART LOCK-IN to send love to each other—perhaps one of the most enjoyable experiences a family can share; it not only increases family coherence and bonding, but it sets the tone of quality time together firmly in a loving, grounded place.

Along with her husband and two young children, Joanne does a brief HEART LOCK-IN before eating dinner every night. "It's like a tonic for the family," Joanne says. "Each of us chooses who we want to send love to. You can feel the energy shift. It's our only real time together. And it makes a huge difference."

Creating a family environment that cultivates core heart feelings and real care between parents and children has to become every parent's priority. Establishing stronger intuitive bonding with one's children is the first step for giving guidance that will be heard—developing respect and easing discipline challenges. Developing skill in emotional management is essential for developing a broader intelligence to successfully deal with the pressures and obstacles that inevitably arise in life.

## HeartMath in Education

Children's values, character, and perceptions of life are also strongly influenced by peers and teachers in the educational environment. One of the most important and rewarding uses of the HeartMath Solution is taking place in classrooms around the country. Currently, 127 teachers and counselors have been officially certified to teach the HeartMath concepts and techniques in their classrooms. In addition, many schools, both private and public, are incorporating HeartMath into their curriculum.

In 1996, Palm Springs Middle School in Dade County, Florida, began a HeartMath intervention program for seventh-grade students. Many of the students spoke Spanish primarily, with English as a second language, and some had difficult home lives. The program aimed to reinforce resiliency skills and positive citizenship while counteracting the effects of stress on learning.

The results were significant. The dedicated schoolteachers, along with Heart-Math staff, saw a definitive shift in all of the key parameters of the Achievement Inventory Measurement used to evaluate the program. As a result of using the HeartMath Solution tools and techniques, the students felt more motivated at school, were more focused in their schoolwork, and felt better able to organize and manage their time, both at school and at home. Their leadership and communication skills improved, and problems with risky or harmful behavior dropped markedly. The students felt more supported by their families and friends, felt more comfortable with themselves and their teachers, and showed increased compassion with their peers. In addition, the students were more assertive and independent in their decision-making, were more resistant to the demands of peer pressure, and were much better able to manage their stress, anger, and negative self-talk. In essence, the students showed increased satisfaction and control over their lives while with friends, at school, and with their families. The graph in Figure 11.1 provides a partial summary of the results.

This program was so successful that in 1997, fifteen of the students from Palm Springs were selected for a cross-age mentoring program at a nearby elementary school, where they tutored fifty-five second- and third-graders in the HeartMath tools and techniques.

Later that year the program was expanded to include two full-year elective courses, called "Heart Smarts," for middle-grade students. The Heart Smarts curriculum offered a series of tools and strategies to help students reduce stress, sustain academic focus, improve communication skills, and enhance peer, teacher, and family relations.

More cross-age mentoring programs are underway at the elementary and middle school levels in Dade County, and these schools plan to make Heart-Math available to more than fifteen hundred students over the next four years. Palm Springs Middle School is also expanding the program to include more

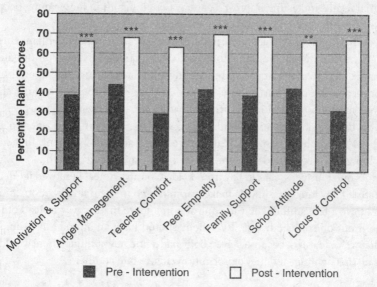

**Achievement Inventory Measurement Scales**

*The Impact of the HeartMath Solution Tools and Techniques on Schoolchildren*

FIGURE 11.1. After learning the HeartMath Solution tools and techniques, a class of seventh-graders in a large metropolitan area showed vast improvements in achievement-related skills, attitudes, and emotional self-management. As a result of practicing the tools, the students' relationships and attitudes toward their schoolwork, their teachers, their friends, their families, and themselves all significantly improved. This graph shows a partial summary of the study's results. \*\*p - .01, \*\*\*p - .001.

© copyright 1998 Institute of HeartMath Research Center

"tracks" after its success teaching FREEZE-FRAME to deaf and hard-of-hearing students. Because many of these students are also language-delayed, they must work two or sometimes three times as hard as their hearing peers, yet they mastered FREEZE-FRAME with considerable enthusiasm.

In conjunction with the work being done in these schools, the Institute of HeartMath is involved with the Miami Heart Research Institute in a study measuring the effects of the HeartMath Solution tools and techniques on the cardiovascular health of middle school students. Preliminary results are showing a marked change in heart rate variability coherence in students practicing Heart-Math (in comparison with students in the control group, who didn't receive training). The final analysis of this study isn't yet available, so stay tuned. The initial results indicating improved cardiovascular health in these young people look more than promising, however.

What better place than our schools to introduce the life skills enhancement that the HeartMath Solution tools and techniques provide. Unfortunately, many of our school systems are burdened with a host of financial, disciplinary, and academic problems. These problems, along with the curriculum challenges that most educators and school boards face, limit their ability to give students the life-skills training they need. Yet the educators in the Dade County school system have demonstrated, with courage and commitment, that such training *can* be provided if the interest and desire are strong enough.

As one fourteen-year-old boy from Dade County wrote, "I enjoyed it [Heart-Math]. They taught us how to make our minds go in the right direction, and, if you have a bad attitude, how to control it in a more mature way instead of taking it out on somebody else. Everybody should have an attitude like some of what we've learned, because if everybody had a fine new attitude, there wouldn't be all this fighting, and they'd probably even love one another."

## How Kids Respond to the Tools of the Heart

When our staff takes the HeartMath Solution tools and techniques into schools across the country, we're able to see the power of the heart in new, inspirational ways. And kids warm to these tools right away. They're so much more inclined to look to their hearts for answers than are adults. Their ability to trust what their hearts tell them shows up in very clear ways.

In the challenging, competitive world of today's young people, a meek, sentimental brand of heart just wouldn't cut it. But these tools help make kids stronger, more self-reliant. When they check in with their hearts, they're empowered to make intelligent choices rather than impulsive ones. And in addition to giving them a sense of care and cooperation, their hearts give them a greater sense of honor.

The school-based discipline of children is also enhanced when they're taught emotional management skills. Teachers who've learned the HeartMath Solution tools and techniques—Judith Carter among them—are saving time and energy by using a method called "time-in." "If I ask a child to do a 'time-in,' it means go do a HEART LOCK-IN and then see if he or she can find a better choice of behavior. It works very well and helps the children manage their emotions," says Carter.

"I have an egg timer in the 'time-in' area of the classroom so the children can time their HEART LOCK-INS. One day, one of the younger students asked me if she could have a 'time-in.' She went to the area, sat down, and did the HEART LOCK-IN with a big smile on her face. I was so proud that she'd managed her own emotions. She told me that she'd taught her daddy how to do a HEART LOCK-IN too."

The tools work especially well during periods of physical activity, such as playground games or sports. Last summer, Beth McNamee, a certified Heart-Math trainer, taught FREEZE-FRAME to sixty children, aged seven through fourteen, at a soccer camp in upstate New York. Once the kids had learned to FREEZE-FRAME, Beth gave them a stressful situation to practice on.

The kids were divided into two teams and asked to kick the soccer ball in a specific pattern. As they practiced the pattern, Beth listened to their remarks: "This is too hard!" "I can't do this!" "Get out of my way!" "You're doing it wrong!" One frustrated team even ganged up on one of their own players and blamed him for throwing everything off.

When the practice ended, Beth asked what they were feeling. One after another, they expressed frustration, anger, defeat, and disappointment with themselves. Even though it was a game, they weren't having any fun.

A few minutes of FREEZE-FRAME helped them refocus in their hearts. Instead of criticizing themselves and one another or trying to place the highest value on getting the pattern perfect, their perspective shifted. In touch with the values of the heart, they took a more amiable, open-minded view.

Suddenly conscious of their injustice, the members of the team that had blamed one boy for their failure apologized and shared the responsibility for their performance. Both groups began to cooperate more freely. Instead of focusing on how they were stuck, they came up with new solutions.

The whole process was more efficient when each team began to work as a unit instead of as a group of separate individuals. The wisdom of their hearts enabled them to be at their best, both as individuals and as a team.

We've found that HeartMath tools and techniques help kids develop skills that will assist them whether they're playing soccer now or competing in the job market of the future. By the use of FREEZE-FRAME alone, they're able to tap into their best assessments. They begin to communicate and get along better with others. By contrast, when they're not in touch with the core values of their hearts, their worlds become at least as frustrating and stressful as the adult world their parents hope to help them avoid.

## Helping Disadvantaged Kids

N othing compares to the disadvantages brought on by lack of genuine love in the crucial developmental years of childhood. Disadvantaged children are most disadvantaged when core heart feelings such as love, care, and appreciation are missing from their family lives. In some inner-city families especially, the family environment can be so challenging that it's hard to see how to help children cultivate core heart feelings.

After conducting a parenting training for inner-city parents, Edie Fritz, a HeartMath educational trainer, reported the following story. A grandmother who was raising her grandchild because the child's parents were unable to, asked, "How can you teach them to appreciate? These kids have so little to appreciate." Edie replied, "Appreciation helps the kids build an inner muscle that strengthens them so that they don't give up so easily. When children stop appreciating, they lose hope. That's when they stop trying and do drugs or join gangs."

Edie then told a story about two of her disadvantaged inner-city students, a boy and a girl, who were struggling to find something (anything) to appreciate about their lives. One day the girl shared that her mother had smiled at her that morning; that was her appreciation. The boy brought a rose to class. He explained that he walked by a rose bush every morning on the way to school. That day the bush had been in bloom; the rose was his appreciation. Edie explained, "Once children open their hearts again to what appreciation is, they begin to find all kinds of little things to appreciate. That's when you start to see major changes in classroom behavior and learning."

For many children, one of the worst stressors in life is being labeled "at-risk" or "disadvantaged," which only adds to feelings of separateness and instability which may be the only constant in their lives. This is especially true for migrant children. As a counselor for the Region X Migrant Education Division of the Los Angeles County Office of Education, Amelia Moreno and a team of credentialed administrators, teachers, and parent mentors serve approximately thirteen thousand migrant families. Their main goal is to help the children (from infancy through age twenty-one) to be successful academically like all other children, despite extreme poverty and mobility and the fact that nearly 100 percent of these kids speak Spanish as their first language.

Working in the areas of agriculture, packing, fishing, and other seasonal jobs, these families don't often stay in one place for more than a few years. Since they move so often, the children can receive a spotty education. Stress can arise for the family as they struggle to keep the more traditional ways of their native cultures and also keep up with the fast-moving American culture.

Amelia uses a Spanish version of HeartMath's curriculum in a migrant "Even Start" family literacy program called "Corazon Contento," or "Happy Heart." Last year (and the previous four years) her program reached three hundred migrant families in fourteen preschool sites around Los Angeles County. As part of this program, preschoolers and their parents attend school together, in adjacent classrooms. While the children are learning kindergarten-readiness skills, their parents are learning English as a second language and working on their literacy and parenting skills. HeartMath plays a pivotal role here, as parents learn FREEZE-FRAME skills with their children, along with other related games and activities from a Spanish translation of the book *Teaching Children to Love*. [9] Amelia says, "Reinforcing the heart values of these families helps them stay on the road to literacy together."

"I've been in education for twenty-eight years now," Amelia explains. "I've found that people need tools to help themselves be successful and to strengthen the efforts of those around them. We want to give our children every indication that they have great potential, limited only by their own beliefs about themselves. So we have to be strong and functional ourselves—to be a model to our families—so they can continue feeling hopeful.

"It's the same in farming as well; you have to prepare the soil. We help the families stay involved in lifelong education by nourishing their intelligence so that it will be fruitful. That's why we use tools that are vital and life-giving. They help us appreciate our rich culture and look forward to the future instead of focusing on what we don't have. The quality of life, the capacity to love and be loved, that light that shines through adversity, these are the qualities that are ultimately most important. In this way, hope serves as the wellspring of life in all cultures."

To improve our society and our world, we have to go back to the basics— back to the family, where the core heart values that make up a world worth living in are meant to be developed and nurtured. If our families are unable to fulfill this role, then our schools, churches, hospitals, businesses, and community-service organizations *must*; it's not a question of *should*. Unless people step in to fulfill the heart-centered nurturing role, we abandon hope of providing a secure foundation for our social future.

To the degree that the HeartMath Solution is able to help individuals, families, children, schools, and communities engage heart intelligence and consider new solutions, it's serving its purpose. As individuals, young and old, develop their heart intelligence, they become the hope for the future.

## KEY POINTS TO REMEMBER

### AT HOME

➤ Do a HEART LOCK-IN with your children at the start of family time, quality time, or before dinner or bed.

➤ When giving instructions, FREEZE-FRAME with your children so that you communicate more coherently and they listen to you better.

➤ If a child is upset, help her do a FREEZE-FRAME or CUT-THRU to calm her emotions.

➤ Teach your children about core heart values and point out to them when they're being appreciative, caring, and nonjudgmental, and when they're not.

➤ Foster emotional management from the heart as often as you can. Use the HeartMath tools and techniques just for the sake of using them and building your family's heart power. The practice will pay off for you and your children in the future.

### AT SCHOOL

➤ Encourage children to go to the heart to solve social conflicts with a more mature perspective. When students are in conflict, promote self-responsibility by asking them to FREEZE-FRAME to find new solutions to resolve their differences.

➤ In any sport activity, call a group FREEZE-FRAME when frustration levels interfere with performance. Use FREEZE-FRAME prior to and after sports activities to clarify goals, increase motivation, and evaluate results.

➤ Use the heart to increase mental clarity and gain wider perspectives in academic subjects. If the students understand heart intelligence, ask them (for example) how historical events might have been different if the people involved had used the HeartMath tools and techniques.

➤ Use a HEART LOCK-IN at the start of the day to prepare students to learn.

➤ Ask children to do a HEART LOCK-IN during "time-ins," to help them balance and manage their emotions.

➤ Have the children do a HEART LOCK-IN after recess if they're overly excited or unable to concentrate.

# CHAPTER 12

# Social Impact

As we begin to experience more care for ourselves and our families, our capacity for the expression of core heart feelings will grow stronger. It's only natural that we'll then look for ways to extend that care into our workplaces and society. But we won't have to become philanthropists or join social causes to affect others with care. As we apply heart intelligence to whatever daily situation we find ourselves in, we'll naturally see new ways to care.

Tom McGuiness, vice president of Mission Effectiveness and Community Outreach for Citrus Valley Health Partners (in California), has always had a vocation for service. Following the impulses of his heart, he's tended to the needs of populations for whom healthcare is neither affordable nor accessible. Long before he was introduced to the tools and techniques of the HeartMath Solution, Tom understood only too well that we live in a world that needs more heart. Like many of those who dedicate their lives to others, Tom feels a strong sense of responsibility to his community and is committed to making it a better place for everyone to live and work.

The lives of dedicated community servants such as Tom contain lessons for us all. With the guidance of heart intelligence, we can find ways to help improve the lives of others. As we increase our internal coherence, we'll experience more intelligent awareness regarding the needs of our communities, and we'll have more energy and inclination to contribute to their well-being.

Our communities are comprised of organizations that impact people's lives. For example, organizations are responsible for the availability and quality of the products we purchase and the services we need, our social infrastructures, our schools, our medical care, and more.

The HeartMath Solution is highly effective at increasing mental and emotional coherence within organizations. The people in organizations who are trained in HeartMath tools and techniques become happier, healthier, and more productive. Customer satisfaction increases. Our communities are strengthened as a result. We've seen some impressive and rewarding results when the Heart-Math Solution has been applied in companies, government agencies, churches, hospitals, and other institutions.

## Corporations

M any companies cope with complex challenges as they struggle to improve profitability through restructuring or repositioning themselves in today's rapidly changing business environment. When restructuring policies are implemented, they often involve abrupt cutbacks with little manifest concern for the people involved. For coherent organizational transformation to take place with the least cost to the company, change initiatives need to be implemented with enough care to reduce the stressful consequences.

Work overload and increased pressure to become more productive are common workplace stressors today. In addition, workers are troubled by uncertainty about their future, longer work hours, decreasing levels of job satisfaction, poor communication, and diminished belief in the organization's loyalty to them. According to the U.S. Department of Labor, the workplace is the greatest single source of stress, no matter what we do or how much we earn. [1]

Without a high degree of emotional management, the increasing pressure of today's workplace takes a large toll on executives and managers, draining away energy at the cost of their personal and family lives. We're seeing more men and women making the choice to take less pay or forego career advancement in exchange for more flexible work hours, reduced pressure, and more time for bonding with their children. For many it comes down to this: What's it worth to be able to run an errand in the middle of the day, go to your son's soccer game, and sleep well at night?

From a business perspective, it isn't always possible to provide flexible work hours, but there's much that companies can do to improve job satisfaction. It doesn't serve the long-term bottom line to treat employees without care and consideration. Time and again, the result of that approach has been a steady decrease in productivity and profitability. Key people become ill or leave, and many who stay become cynical and unmotivated in an uncaring work environment.

Conversely, those companies that care enough to give people the skills and opportunities to more efficiently manage their work and lives gain loyal employees with a greater ability to adapt and remain enthusiastic. They become more resilient and creative amid change. Performance improves. It's a good business investment to allot resources toward fostering work/life balance and mental/emotional self-management in the corporate setting.

In 1998 the *Wall Street Journal* reported on a study conducted by Sears & Roebuck. At eight hundred stores, the results showed that happy employees not only stayed with the company; they also generated free word-of-mouth advertising by recommending company products to others. When employee attitudes improved by a mere 5 percent, Sears found that customer satisfaction jumped 1.3 percent. This resulted in a 0.5 percent rise in revenue—a substantial gain for a corporation of that size.

"We know employee satisfaction does increase customer satisfaction, as well as productivity," Brian McQuaid, executive director of MCI, reported in the same article. But furthermore, at MCI, even a 5 percent drop in employee efficiency cuts annual revenue by "a couple of hundred million dollars." It's only good business sense to keep employees satisfied and doing their best in a corporate environment. [2]

Now, and especially in the near future, more and more companies will rise or fall based on the collective inner quality of their employees. The days of the indifferent corporate machine are over. Those companies that realize this and take appropriate action will be the most likely to grow and prosper in the new millennium.

## Heart in the Workplace

At first glance, it might seem as if attention to the heart would be somewhat out of place in the business environment. The belief that "business is business" and emotion has no place in the workplace is still prevalent in many circles. Amazing as it seems, it's not uncommon for our trainers to hear executives complain that they don't need "soft" skills.

But for the most part, HeartMath's pragmatic view of the heart—combined as it is with biomedical support and a results-driven process—is met with great receptivity by corporations. When core heart values and new methods that increase heart intelligence are brought into the workplace, positive change occurs quickly and dramatically.

Bruce Cryer, the vice president of Global Business Development for Heart-Math LLC, teaches heart-based skills with corporations nationwide and has witnessed the impact of those skills firsthand. To Bruce, the need for heart in a corporation makes perfect sense. "Consider that all organizations are living systems composed of people who think and feel," Bruce says. "Each organization really is a large, complex organism whose health and resilience depends on many of the same factors that determine an individual's health and balance. Smart organizations—like smart people—will recognize and seek to measure the elements that are working as well as those that are out of balance." [3]

In 1994, Bruce took his team into Motorola with the goal of enhancing employee performance. The company already had a global reputation for product innovation, in part because it devoted unusually strong attention to the needs of its people. But increased competition had raised the stakes. Stress was higher than usual. In typical Motorola form, the management was concerned and took action.

The HeartMath team was asked to address the issues of productivity, teamwork, communication skills, stress, health, creativity, and innovation. Bruce and his team taught the HeartMath Solution to Motorola employees and did assessments both before and after to measure any changes. After six months of practicing the tools and techniques of HeartMath, participants showed a dramatic difference in their performance.

- 93 percent had increased productivity.
- 90 percent had improved teamwork.
- 93 percent felt a greater sense of empowerment.
- 93 percent felt healthier.

Assembly-line workers—who were among the employee groups trained—reported significantly more energy and vitality. They felt less tension and noticed fewer physical problems during the six-month period, and they felt greater personal and professional fulfillment in their work by the end of that time.

Motorola was also interested in the relationship between their employees' cardiovascular health and their efficiency at work. The company was aware that 28 percent of American adults have high blood pressure. Not only is that health problem the leading risk factor for heart disease and stroke, but it can also significantly inhibit performance and productivity.

Although the HeartMath team focused on increasing the productivity of the company, the reduction in tension and stress generated clear health benefits as well. At the beginning of the six-month period, 28 percent of the workers on the executive, administrative, and engineering teams had high blood pressure, in keeping with the national average. Afterwards, everyone who practiced the HeartMath Solution tools and techniques had regained normal blood pressure readings! [4]

The lowered experience of stress was experienced both objectively and subjectively. One employee said, "I'm handling family life a lot better with fewer worries and I've resolved a lot of prolonged issues. I can listen to others, be open-minded, be willing to train co-workers, and come to work feeling happy and ready to work."

Participants in the program reported a reduction in anxiety (18 percent), burnout (26 percent), and hostility (20 percent), along with an increase in contentment (32 percent). Overall, they achieved a 36 percent reduction in stress symptoms, including sleeplessness, rapid heartbeats, headaches, heartburn, and trembling.

Since that time, more than a thousand Motorola employees have gone through the HeartMath corporate training program with similar results, and this course has been adopted as the primary stress management program at Motorola University in Schaumburg, Illinois. Motorola's experience has proved that tapping into the intelligence of the heart can directly impact a corporation's bottom line.

## Applying Heart to Corporations

When we take the HeartMath Solution into the corporate arena, we use a program called "Inner Quality Management" (IQM). The same basic tools and techniques that you've learned in this book, along with several more, are directed toward four specific objectives:

- Improving internal self-management
- Achieving coherent communication
- Boosting organizational climate
- Facilitating strategic processes and renewal

Internal self-management provides a new foundation for individual effectiveness and productivity. Coherent communication plays a vital role in team-building. A constructive and supportive organizational climate provides fertile ground for a thriving operation in the long term. Strategic renewal keeps the whole operation invigorated and ensures that the company's resources will be continually replenished.

To help companies achieve these objectives, HeartMath trainers teach FREEZE-FRAME as a means to reduce stress and increase mental clarity. Employees learn to evaluate their energy assets and deficits. In advanced courses, CUT-THRU is introduced to further improve emotional balance. To regenerate before or after work or during breaks, many employees make use of the HEART LOCK-IN technique as well.

At Royal Dutch Shell in the United Kingdom, HeartMath consultants trained 150 middle- and senior-level managers and observed significant improvements—especially in the group with the highest stress levels. There were reductions of 65 percent in tension, 87 percent in fatigue, 65 percent in anger, and 44 percent in intentions to leave the company. These major changes took place in just six weeks. To determine the retention value of the HeartMath tools and techniques, the consultants went back after six months for further assessment. The participants had had more time to perfect their skills, and the results showed it. In every area tested, the indicators of stress had continued to decrease.

These studies illustrate just how powerful developing heart coherence at work can be. Most of us spend a large percentage of our time at work, and all of us in some way interact with companies and depend on their products and services. As executives and managers recognize the practical benefits of heart intelligence in the workplace, and encourage its development, they'll provide a tremendous service to their shareholders, employees, customers, and communities.

## Government Agencies

For many years, Joseph Sundram, director of HeartMath's Organizational Programs Division, has taken our programs to remarkably diverse branches of the government. This experience offers him an unusual window of opportunity to see what happens when the HeartMath Solution is applied by civil servants, military personnel, police officers in high-risk encounters, and others who serve in the infrastructures of local, state, and federal government organizations.

Government employees face many of the same stresses and challenges as their private-sector counterparts. But they also face challenges unique to the public sector.

From the start, government work offered employees something that has now almost vanished from the private sector—the security of lifelong employment if employees played by the rules. To prevent management by whim, civil service rules and regulations set the parameters for fair practices in employment, promotion, and dismissal. But if you ask managers how these rules *really* are applied, their frustration level may skyrocket. One of the unintended consequences of the rules has been the difficulty in getting rid of people who are no longer doing an acceptable job.

"In a corporation, if you consistently do your job poorly you get fired," Joseph explains. "With civil service protections, if someone consistently does his or her job poorly, it may still take two or three years to remove that person from a position. Often the problem individual is simply transferred, becoming some other government organization's problem."

Unlike corporations, many government agencies are single-source monopolies. This creates a distinctive mind-set among some civil servants. With a disproportionate value placed on the status quo, the heart qualities of care, flexibility, and excellence can become irrelevant. In most cases, it's the rigidity of the system itself and the uncaring excesses of a few individuals that tarnish the quality of service for many.

In government agencies, change is necessarily subject to the slowly turning gears of a sluggish bureaucracy, but the profound changes that have already taken place are challenging the security that government workers have always depended on. Military bases have downsized or closed; the expectation of life-long service in the military can no longer be taken for granted. As the armed forces become leaner and more technology-based, fewer, more versatile, and better-educated people have a good shot at a full career. In recent years, thousands in the military have been forced to find new careers.

But according to Joseph, even before these outside pressures came to bear, many government agencies knew that they had to change. The information explosion was requiring new technologies and skills to move from a paper-based environment to more efficient computer-based information management systems. Morale problems were on the rise. Customer service complaints were piling up. The lack of care was taking as high a toll on the employees and organizations as it was on the customers themselves.

Consider the challenge that faced a Canadian utility company that generates and distributes electrical power for much of North America. When electrical power was deregulated in the United States, this Canadian entity was forced to redesign itself in order to be competitive and to survive. If it couldn't change adequately, it would lose its life in the marketplace—and lose tens of thousands of jobs, as well as national and regional pride.

Founded and operated for decades as a public company, it was recently "de-merged" into three public and private companies. Long-standing ways of doing business and serving customers—even the core identity as a government entity—had to change. Employees, once secure in their future as part of a government-owned monopoly, had to learn the language of cost effectiveness, competition, and customer care. The message was clear: change or perish.

It hasn't been an easy transition. A 1998 study conducted by the Institute of HeartMath showed profound changes in attitude, performance, and health in an experimental group who received the Inner Quality Management program (when compared to a control group who received no training). Psychological tests were administered just prior to the one-day training and then again twelve weeks after.

Sleeplessness increased by 15 percent in the control group but dropped by 11 percent in the experimental group. Social support (as evidenced by a sense of collegiality with co-workers) improved by 13 percent among the experimental group compared to a rise of just 3 percent in the control group. Anxiety dropped by 13 percent in the experimental group compared to a drop of just 3 percent in the control group. Job satisfaction improved by 13 percent in the experimental group compared to a drop of 1 percent in the control group. Productivity dropped by 5 percent in the control group during this turbulent time but managed a 1 percent increase in the experimental group. (See Figure 12.1.)

The implications of these results are much greater than just putting employees in a good mood. As Joseph points out, "Care is a lubricant at the biological, cognitive, organizational, and service levels. Entrained organizations made up of entrained individuals generate more effective and efficient systems. They learn faster and deeper, and they're more able to be flexible as the requirements of the job change. They experience greater fulfillment from truly being of service to themselves, their colleagues, and others." Because government agencies were designed for public service, entrainment brings both the individuals and the organization into closer alignment with their mission.

We work with many government agencies and corporations, and it's encouraging to see data that illustrates a consistent pattern of improvement in the physical and emotional well-being of the employees we've had the opportunity to train. This underscores our belief in the effectiveness of heart intelligence to overcome challenges individually and collectively.

## The Urban Battlefield

People who work in corporations or government agencies face many challenges and stressful situations, but no group of people faces as much

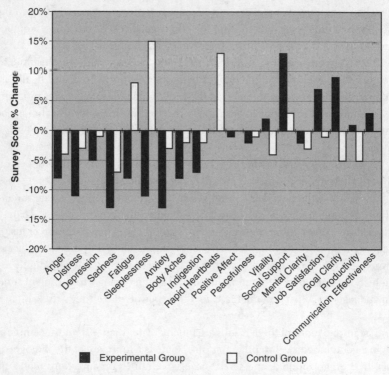

**Experimental Group**     ☐ **Control Group**

*The Impact of the HeartMath Solution Tools and Techniques on Organizational Health and Effectiveness*

FIGURE 12.1. During a turbulent organizational transition, employees of a large Canadian utility company who were trained in the HeartMath Solution tools and techniques showed improvements in emotional balance, physical health, and work effectiveness (black bars). A control group who didn't use the tools showed opposite trends in many of these areas (white bars).

© copyright 1998 Institute of HeartMath Research Center

potential for stress as those who serve in law enforcement. On our own city streets, police officers work in a war zone. Putting their lives at risk is a core facet of their job. It's not surprising that police officers have one of the worst records of any profession for forced retirement, catastrophic illness, and early death. On a daily basis, they experience the nonstop accumulation of both minor and extreme stresses. The accusations of police brutality among a small group of officers in recent years seem almost inevitable in the context of such high-stress work.

Imagine that you're a police officer. All day long you've encountered one hostile, potentially life-threatening situation after another. Near the end of your shift, when you try to stop someone for speeding, he flees. Then you chase the driver for forty-five minutes, adrenaline pumping into your system constantly. Trying to recalibrate your biological fight-or-flight response after a day like that, so that you can act appropriately in the "civilian" world you head home to, takes an exceptional level of self-management.

Now think about the car chase again. If you succumb to feelings of rage and hostility in that stressful situation, your physical coordination will be heightened, but desynchronization of your mental processes will take place. As a result, the function of the cortex—that part of the brain that allows you to make decisions of all kinds, including moral choices—will be impaired. In the heat of such a moment, the more primitive regions of the brain are hard at work. [5] Without the mitigating impulses of the more complex regions of the brain, you might see it as perfectly natural to yank the suspect from his car and beat him to a pulp.

Shifting to the heart before dealing with the suspect would give you a tremendous advantage. You'd be able to disengage from some of the anger, frustration, and blame you felt during the chase and come from a place that's more objective and neutral. Your mental clarity and decision-making ability would increase and your reaction speed and coordination improve. Then, even if the situation called for the use of force, you'd be able to apply the appropriate level of force for the particular situation. Too much force could harm the suspect, the case, and your career, and it could even cause a community-wide conflagration; too little could jeopardize safety and lead to injury or death for innocent bystanders, yourself, and your colleagues. With your heart involved in decision-making, your biology would be in sync with its best ability to function, and you'd be able to see your actions in a larger perspective.

In a 1998 study sponsored by seven police chiefs, the Institute of HeartMath followed officers from seven different police departments in a large metropolitan area through an exercise called a "scenario"—a simulated police call conducted while carrying munitions incapable of injuring the officers and participants.

Outside a specially designed warehouse facility police officers are briefed about the scenario. They're told that a possible breaking-and-entering has occurred. A usually secure door standing ajar supports the suspicion of trouble. There may or may not be people still inside; if there are, it's unknown whether they're employees or criminals (or both). They may or may not be armed. Figure 12.2 shows the physiological reaction of a single officer going through the simulation.

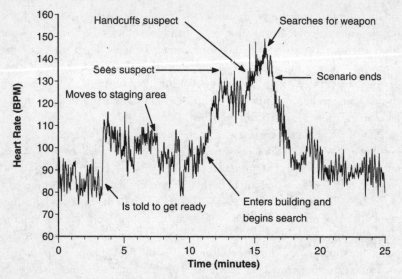

*Heart Rhythm of a Police Officer During a Simulated Police Call*

FIGURE 12.2. This graph shows the heart rate variability of a police officer during a simulated search of a warehouse for a suspect who may be armed. Note the rapid and large increase in the officer's heart rate when he enters the building. He thinks that the suspect has a hidden weapon and attempts to search for it, but he can't find it. His heart rate reaches a maximum at this point. Later, the officer will report this to be the most stressful part of the scenario.

© copyright 1998 Institute of HeartMath Research Center

Although the officer knows that this is only a simulation, we can see clear beginnings of the fight-or-flight response even as he's being told to get ready. His heart rate begins to rise, and its rhythms become disordered. Once he moves to the staging area (where he's briefed and makes final preparations), there's another jolt from his stimulated sympathetic nervous system, causing a spike in his heart rhythms, as his heart rate rises even more. Pulling his weapon, he warily enters the building, scanning the boxes and materials stacked around the room for potential hiding places. As he does so, his heart rate jumps again. His heart is now beating faster than two beats a second.

Suddenly he sees someone in a far corner of the room. He barks out, "Police! Raise your hands and come out!" By this time, his heart is beating nearly three times a second (the rhythm very jagged), his blood pressure has soared, and adrenaline and cortisol are coursing through his system. This is no longer make-believe to his body.

In the confusing seconds that follow, the intruder claims to be an employee and reaches inside his jacket for identification. The police officer's voice is shrill and insistent in his continuing commands: "Down on the ground! Now! Do it!" In the next minute or so, the officer brings the suspect under control by handcuffing him. There the simulation ends.

As you can see in the graph, this simulation caused a massive fight-or-flight response. There's a fairly quick drop from this state to the first stage of recalibration, but it takes ten or more minutes for the officer to really come down from the experience. During that time, his heart is still racing. Even after it's all over, he leaves the simulation with a higher pulse than when he began.

One of the reasons that seven chiefs of police have sponsored joint Heart-Math trainings for their officers in seventy offices is to achieve the considerable benefit that HeartMath tools and techniques have on performance in the high-stress situations that police work involves. Another is to help officers recalibrate quickly in the field.

But there's another, more personal reason that these organizations are using the HeartMath Solution to develop the skills of the heart. After spending eight hours or more dealing with some of the less pleasant aspects of society, it's extremely hard for an officer to leave those experiences behind and go home to be a loving father/mother, husband/wife, or son/daughter. Sometimes officers respond to accidents or crime scenes where people have suffered grue-some, untimely deaths. These images and the feelings they engender must be muted or suppressed to get the job done in the moment. But such scenes can haunt officers for a long time afterwards. Learning to keep their perspective in balance, even when confronting the darker sides of human behavior, is no small feat.

The HeartMath Solution gives police officers, and anyone else involved in high-stress work, the tools needed to let go of stress and return to the heart at will. People who use these skills in moments of crisis are more likely to perform at their peak at a time when they need all the resources they can muster.

The HeartMath Police Study has shown that the tools and techniques of the HeartMath Solution can make a significant difference in the lives of police offi-cers in a variety of policing functions. Thirty officers in an experimental group received three sessions of HeartMath training over a four-week period, while a control group of thirty officers received no training during the same period.

They were tested before the program began and again four weeks after the training ended.

As Figure 12.3 shows, depression increased among the control group by 17 percent over a sixteen-week period. During the same period, depression declined among trained officers by 13 percent. Among the control group, distress dropped by 1 percent, while the experimental group experienced a 20 percent decline in stress. Fatigue declined among the trained group by 18 percent, while those not trained in HeartMath had a decline of only 1 percent.

The men and women of our police departments make great sacrifices to serve our communities and nation. Providing them with skills to perform their jobs with the least amount of stress and suffering, and to shift gears between emotional states more easily, allows them to serve effectively and then enjoy focused time with their families when they go home each day. It also prevents the slow and deadly accumulation of stress that leads to the unusually high rates of cardiovascular disease and post-retirement mortality known to exist among officers. They deserve more for their selfless service. Learning to use their heart intelligence can help them enjoy the coherent flow of a quality life.

## Serving Others

One of the primary reasons that HeartMath training works so effectively in many different types of organizations is that organizations are composed of individuals working together. It's through improving our cooperative efforts that heart intelligence will have the most impact on society.

The best thing any one of us can do for society is to start with ourselves first. By living from the heart effectively, we set an example that encourages others around us to want the same for themselves. As you listen to your heart, its intuitive voice will provide the insight and guidance you need to assist them.

One key to determining how best to express your heart intelligence in service to others is to always distinguish between care and overcare when deciding what and how much to do. Many good intentions have fallen short of the intended mark by allowing overcare to drain away energy in the name of care. It's important not to let good intentions get in the way of doing what's most effective. Use heart discrimination, not an overexcited head, to decide where to invest time and energy.

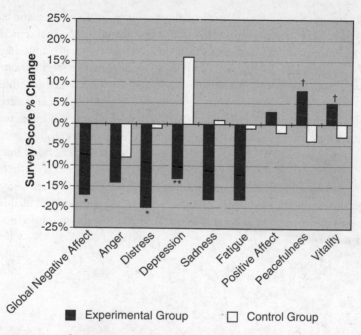

*Improvements in Stress Levels in Police Officers Practicing the HeartMath Solution Tools and Techniques*

FIGURE 12.3. Police officers who practiced the tools and techniques of the HeartMath Solution showed significant reductions in stress, negative emotions, and physical stress symptoms (black bars). Results are compared to a control group not trained in the tools (white bars) $+<1$, $*$ $p< .05$, $**$ $p< .01$.

© copyright 1998 Institute of HeartMath Research Center

As heart intelligence is refined, it leads to a mature understanding of what service is. It's still all about love—but love with a practical bottom line that understands the most efficient use of energy.

As you continue to practice the HeartMath tools and techniques, accumulating energy assets and eliminating energy deficits, you'll build not only a more refined sense of service but also the power to effect productive change in the areas where you choose to serve. Go for deepening your connection with your own heart first, and opportunities to share your heart with others in meaningful ways will find you.

Throughout this book we've presented practical tools, techniques, and concepts you can use to improve your life. We've also shared biomedical research, personal stories, and organizational applications to provide greater understanding of the power and intelligence of the heart. In the final chapter we depart somewhat from this theme. We offer you a view of how we perceive the current state of our world, the future of heart intelligence, and a theoretical model of how the development of individual and collective coherence will impact present and future events. Chapter 13 is intended to promote a consideration of exciting, new possibilities and a broader view of the potential of heart intelligence.

What's most important, however, is that to achieve these possibilities, you make a sincere effort now to apply what you've learned in the previous chapters. As we said in Chapter 1, the last step in the HeartMath Solution is to *actualize what you know.*

# The 21st-Century Heart

In working with people from many different areas of society—including businesses, schools, law enforcement agencies, the medical community, and governmental organizations—we've gained a fairly comprehensive view of the challenges people face. Most people seem to feel overloaded in the present and uncertain about the future. So many changes are occurring simultaneously that it's hard to get a grip on where it's all going. The following story from a senior manager of a large computer company who attended one of our seminars illustrates the uncertainty.

"Our company is going through a merger with another company. Mergers and acquisitions between companies demand a consolidation of resources and technology. It's very stressful for the employees, because you have to work twice as hard doing your own job along with all the other work that comes from merging with people from a different corporate culture with different ways of doing things. You often don't know where you stand. You could get a new supervisor, your position might be eliminated, you could get transferred to a new department or location, or you could get laid off.

"On top of all that, our company is having to respond to the world's Y2K computer problem at the same time. Billions of dollars worth of fairly new computers are getting scrapped because there aren't enough software experts to make them Y2K-compliant. This is costing companies so much that their share values are starting to drop. Our customers are ordering new Y2K-compliant computer systems, but we can't manufacture enough to fill all the orders before the year 2000. Everyone's racing against the clock. The problem is even worse because the government has preempted a lot of the orders that other customers placed so that essential government computers will be Y2K-compliant. In addition to all of that, we're dealing with the Asian economic crisis, and no one knows where the global economy is going. Just trying to keep up with the demands at work is stressful enough, but when I look into the future, I wonder whether what I'm doing is going to make any difference."

The world is indeed in an important transitional era. Technological advancement, globalization in business, and globalization in the media and through the Internet are taking us rapidly into unprecedented opportunities and challenges. We're in a period of high-speed transformation, and everything and everybody is affected by it.

Computerized systems throughout the world, from communications satellites to cell phones to banking transactions, are increasingly interlinked and interdependent. A problem in one area can cause a chain reaction throughout the world. We've all heard potential scenarios that frighten even the most staid among us. As a highly connected global society, we're moving rapidly toward having to make important choices that will affect our present security and the lives of future generations. The world's problems could get worse before they get better. But the very challenges of this time period also present opportunities for a significant shift in human consciousness.

We've entered a developmental phase that heightens the importance of advancing new, intelligent solutions that will promote coherence and alignment rather than division and strife. We at HeartMath see the cultivation of heart intelligence, which exists within all people but lies largely dormant, as our richest resource for achieving this coherence.

## The Global Stress Momentum

The collective energy generated from the feelings, thoughts, and attitudes of the almost six billion people on this planet creates an atmosphere, or "consciousness climate." Surrounding us like the air we breathe, this consciousness climate affects us most strongly on energetic and emotional levels.

An increase in *coherent* thoughts and feelings creates an *uplifting* momentum in the consciousness climate. An increase in *incoherent* thoughts and feelings creates a *stress* momentum in the consciousness climate. In other words, coherence or incoherence is broadcast via the consciousness climate much as music or noise is broadcast via radio signals.

The collective stress that people everywhere are experiencing creates a far-reaching broadcast of internal noise and static. Stress first gets broadcast person to person—in homes, schools, offices, and streets. Then, amplified and reinforced through TV, radio, and print media, the stress momentum goes global, reaching billions of people daily.

When events such as a terrorist bombing that kills hundreds, renewed war-posturing by Saddam Hussein, or nuclear testing in India and Pakistan take place, people all over the world are affected. They feel the tension wave of those unstable situations even though they're not directly impacted. A similar wave is felt following reports of devastating natural disasters, such as earthquakes, floods, hurricanes, or fires.

In quantum physics, there's proof that information can be exchanged almost instantly through what's called "quantum nonlocality." Physicists have done experiments showing that once two particles touch, they remain forever interconnected in some way. Change one particle, and the other one—now miles away—changes simultaneously. When we hear broadcasts on TV that impact our thoughts and moods, we remain connected to that information.

In their book *The Undivided Universe,* quantum physicists David Bohm and Basil Hiley describe this nonlocal connection that unites distant objects. They state, "It takes only a little reflection to see that [this] . . . will apply even more directly and obviously to consciousness, with its constant flow of evanescent thoughts, feelings, desires, urges and impulses. All of these flow into and out of each other." [1] What they have in common is actually a quality of unbroken wholeness.

What these physicists are suggesting is that people's thoughts and emotions are far more interconnected than previously thought. Our propensity toward judgments, projections, overcare, unmanaged emotions, and inflexible mind-sets has created a consciousness climate that's entraining people into a state of incoherence.

As stress waves are generated, our emotions pick up this incoherent energy. Even after the wave passes through, the emotional aftereffects keep reverberating. If you've ever lived through an earthquake and its aftershocks, you may have felt static energy reverberating in your body for days. Strong waves of emotional stress can affect the whole world in a similar way. When events take place that cause massive fear and anxiety, we *all* experience the stress at some level. At the level of consciousness, we're all in this together.

When we look at the physics of collective consciousness, the nature of incoherence and coherence becomes increasingly important. Our own emotional management also ranks high on the priority list. Depending on how self-managed we are, we can deflect some of this stress influence. However, we can still be vulnerable to increases in the stress frequency in the world around us—increases that amplify our mental overprocessing and emotional reactivity and push us past our tolerance threshold.

## The Coherence Momentum

The global stress momentum is obvious, but there's an equally potent force opposing it. Even as the waves of stress and incoherence increase, the energetics of coherence—the other side of living in this era of change—is working in our favor.

Amidst the burgeoning stress, a new momentum toward coherence is building. But we can attune to it and actualize it only through emotional management and balance—skills that much of society lacks. If we stay locked in anxiety, fear, resignation, or an unwillingness to change, the ever-accelerating pace of these times will continue to provide one challenge after another. Finding the heart momentum within is the best way to help ourselves and others navigate through this transitional era.

While there's more incoherence than coherence being transmitted in the mass consciousness at this time, we see considerable evidence of the coherence momentum. More and more people are talking to each other about heart, following their heart, and trying to increase their appreciation, compassion, and personal balance. Bestselling books such as *Don't Sweat the Small Stuff* (by Richard Carlson) and *Simple Abundance* (by Sarah Ban Breathnach) remind us to find gratitude and joy in life.

Many people are experiencing a change in their priorities and values. They've had enough of living a life of ambition and basic survival. An increasing interest in spirituality and religious practices of all kinds illustrates that people are looking for something more. They're seeking, going within themselves the best they know how, looking for meaning and purpose in their lives. All of these examples represent a longing for more heart and for a connection with spirit.

Any time one person makes an effort to contact a deeper part of him- or herself, balance his or her emotions, and deflect the stress momentum, others benefit. As more individuals learn to maintain their poise and balance and refrain from adding to the incoherence around them, they help to counterbalance the frequency of stress. This makes it easier for still others to surf the waves of change instead of being beaten down by them. This coherence momentum makes it easier for new awareness and new solutions for social challenges to emerge globally.

Humanity has reached a point in evolution where heart intelligence is essential. In the near future, emotional management won't seem as much of an *option* as it does now; it will be a *staple*. Engaging heart intelligence facilitates emotional management and aligns us with the coherence momentum. On the strength of that capability, heart intelligence will lead us to the new solutions we need to deal with global challenges. It will also reveal to us our inner technology—the cybernetics of our thoughts and feelings.

Through our experience with heart intelligence, we predict that advances in inner technology will happen even more rapidly in coming years than advances in outer technology did in the last hundred years. We know that's a big statement. But it doesn't just come out of nowhere; it's based on the fact that coherence is more highly organized and powerful than incoherence. Remember, the coherent power of a laser is far more powerful than incandescent light. Incoherence in the human system creates stress and disorder. Society has had enough of that. It's time to explore the potential of coherence.

The transition into heart intelligence will be more significant than the transition from the Middle Ages to the Renaissance and Scientific Revolution, or the transition from the Industrial Revolution to the Information Age of the past century. It represents a dimensional shift in human awareness—and it's already started.

## Science and Spirit

M any ancient forms of medicine considered the body to a have vitalistic spirit, life force, or guiding field. Chinese medicine uses the term *chi* to describe the life force that flows through each person. Vitalistic theories maintain that some nonphysical force or field must be added to the laws of physics and chemistry before we can fully understand life. [2]

The vitalist component has been revived by a number of modern scientists, including Rupert Sheldrake, who postulates the existence of nonphysical, guiding morphogenetic fields, or "form-generating" fields. [3] These nonphysical fields help to explain why many methods of alternative medicine, including prayer, can work. Subtle energy or nonphysical fields of some type appear to be involved, even though science doesn't have instruments sensitive enough to measure them.

The explosive growth of the alternative health movement in the United States and other Western countries in the past decade occurred because people demanded new approaches. They read news reports or saw friends being helped by alternative healing methods and intuitively felt that these methods had much to offer. For years, the National Institutes of Health (NIH) and other medical organizations discounted alternative approaches such as acupuncture and energy healing as unprovable and therefore invalid. Yet NIH was finally forced by Congress to address this field, because millions of people were eschewing traditional medicine and seeking alternative treatments with great benefit. Now NIH has funded an Office of Alternative Medicine to research and identify those alternative approaches that are the most effective (even if those approaches can't yet be scientifically explained).

In the physics community, there's discussion of a "pre-space" from which the physical world, including time and space, is manifest. [1] Physicist Roger Penrose has proposed that the universe is a dynamic spiderweb of quantum spins. These spin networks create an evolving array of tiny geometric volumes that define and inform space-time. [4] Penrose is now collaborating with Stuart Hameroff, a physician, in hopes of finding out how spin networks inform living biological systems. Hameroff introduced the concept of *quantum vitalism*, which views life as derived from and intimately linked to organizing processes at the most fundamental level of the universe. [5] These two men hope to be able to explain scientifically how consciousness and biology (or what some would call *spirit* and *matter*) come together.

It's our view that scientific explanations for subtle energy or form-generating fields will be found as scientists investigate the intelligence and other attributes of the heart. The Institute of HeartMath's research has shown that the electromagnetic field of the heart extends beyond the body. As yet, instruments can measure the heart's field no more than eight to ten feet away from the body, but indications are that it's a nonlocal field that transcends time and space. Physicists William Gough and Robert Shacklett [6], as well as William Tiller [7], have proposed models that connect electromagnetic theory with an inherently nonlinear, nonlocal multidimensional domain that operates under holographic principles. These models, although not yet proven, help explain how the heart's field could extend for miles and possibly across the world.

Based on HeartMath findings indicating that coherence starts in the heart rhythms and is then communicated to the brain and body, it's our theory that the heart is a major conduit through which spirit enters the human system. The qualities of spirit—love, compassion, care, appreciation, tolerance, and patience—all create increased coherence and order in the heart rhythm patterns. Anger, frustration, anxiety, fear, worry, and hostility all create incoherence and disorder in the heart rhythm patterns. As people shift into more coherent heart rhythms, their higher heart intelligence manifests. Their perspective becomes more beneficent and more aware of the whole. From our view, coherence manifests when spirit merges with humanness.

People don't have to wait for science to prove the existence of consciousness or spirit before they start to connect with the organizing intelligence of their heart. Our global society can shift into a new coherent dimension of life experience as sufficient numbers of people make even small efforts to engage the power of the heart with consistency. These efforts will result in a shift from a focus on the mind to a focus on the heart. Each person has to make the choice to shift, but the payoff can be substantial. As more people choose the heart, they'll attune to the heart frequency of others who are doing the same. This will help them ride the waves of the stress momentum and global changes with new ease and grace.

## Societal Coherence

Indicators of increasing social coherence can be seen in the emergence of support groups in record numbers. Whether they're formed by people who share common challenges or people who share common personal-improvement or study goals, these small groups serve as extended families. They provide heart connection and a strengthening of emotional and social support. Support groups help people destress from problems at work and at home. The care that group members exchange while together and each member's individual, at-home efforts to go to the heart help contribute to the wave of coherent consciousness that fosters cooperation and helps buffer people from stress and emotional turmoil.

Even the global stress momentum has its upside. Stress often forces people to go to their hearts for solutions, and it can bring people together. When local crises occur, we set aside racial, cultural, and economic differences and work together for the good of the whole—at least for awhile. Afterwards, we often remember those heartfelt experiences as high points in our lives.

Our experiments on the electricity of touch, mentioned in Chapter 8, proved that our heart's electrical signal shows up in the brain waves of people we touch or who are in close proximity. HeartMath experiments have also shown that the electromagnetic energy produced by the heart radiates outside the body. As we put out more love, care, and appreciation, the heart broadcasts a frequency or wave among people that makes it easier for others to engage with their hearts.

Appreciation alone is a powerful coherence frequency. Appreciation actually amplifies coherence and aligns us with our true selves. It connects us with the planetary heart and our deeper purpose. By actualizing heart qualities in our lives—appreciation, care, compassion, and love—we help propel the coherence momentum in the consciousness field of the planet.

We foresee the coherence momentum eventually reaching critical mass and creating a millennium of peace and prosperity based on new intelligence. Humanity will eventually make the polarity shift from incoherence to coherence. This will allow people everywhere to more easily perceive and act in ways that are individually and collectively balanced and caring.

## Personal Responsibility

As the global accumulation of stress increases, it's easy for emotional distortion to slip up on us in the form of mental overload and emotional reactivity. Overload keeps all of us—rich or poor, educated or uneducated—imprisoned in overidentity with all that's going on. It's a sleep state that perpetuates survival-level living.

In taking personal responsibility, it's important to develop emotional balance and try not to add to the stress momentum. Overcare won't help. Take the challenge and go for maintaining emotional stability in the face of change. Don't cave in. We can all get past feelings of confusion and overload and find a new point of integrity inside ourselves by managing the mind and emotions with heart. This process generates hope and provides access to more of our spirit.

It's not as hard as it used to be to shift to heart coherence. In fact, never before has coherence been so readily accessible, because more and more people are turning to the heart. As a result, our ability to move beyond limitations and experience fulfillment has increased significantly. As we practice following the heart, we'll develop the capabilities and insights we need to address personal and social issues.

There's much insight to be gained during these times by aligning heart and mind. As we achieve alignment, the experience of new awareness will become tangible and alive. Now is the time to take that promise to heart. But *having* insights is different than *acting on them*. We must *follow* the heart and shape a better world for ourselves and the collective whole.

## Change Management—Developing Self-Security

My (Doc's) intent has always been to help people love each other more and experience the source of love and security in their hearts. The HeartMath Solution isn't the only approach to actualizing the heart's potential, but (as we've demonstrated through the work we've done in a variety of social contexts) it works.

The HeartMath Solution tools and techniques cultivate hope. As people develop their own heart intelligence, new hope emerges from within—hope that they can experience peace, happiness, and satisfaction in their lives; hope that they won't get caught up in the stress momentum, that instead they'll make a valuable contribution to the emergence of heart intelligence. But hope can be obscured by chaos. Try to remember that when things appear to be chaotic, it's often because they're in the process of reshaping and transforming for the better.

Guard against the tendency to expect immediate results, especially when dealing with long-standing mental and emotional issues. Often we make a half-hearted effort, then get disappointed when everything isn't instantly okay. Through the heart, mental and emotional distortion can be transmuted in a short period of time; but let's be honest—there are no quick fixes. Certainly the HeartMath Solution isn't a quick fix. It is, however, a process that can fix things quickly when approached with sincerity.

Don't fall into the trap of feeling as if things will never get better or telling yourself, "I've tried, but it's just not working." That period between making an effort to change and actually registering the results is when most people stumble, lapsing back into old behaviors.

When applying any part of the HeartMath Solution, *be patient in your practice*. Don't expect miracles overnight. Try being as consistent as you can in applying these concepts and techniques, and the benefits will find you in due time.

## In the New Days

One thing is for sure: once you make your own paradigm shift from the head to the heart, life will be a lot more fun. That shift is a steady process that alters your internal state step by step. As you make changes in perception and attitude, your outer life will begin to respond accordingly, and increased fulfillment will be the reward.

Fulfillment takes place on the inside first. It's a *feeling* you have. Sure, external gains are part of a person's fulfillment package, but the externals aren't what provides lasting satisfaction. The world is full of people who thought that being rich would bring them fulfillment—only to find that even with huge sums of money their lives were still miserable.

The doorway to fulfillment is in your heart. When you use your heart intelligence to shift perception and direct the flow of your emotions, you have the ability to generate and magnetize your own fulfillment. The longing stops and is replaced by appreciation.

Once you stabilize the connection with your heart intelligence, you'll have more security and freedom to think, feel, and live in ways appropriate for you. A new maturity will allow you to make choices—without fear—that you know are right for you while still sensitively respecting others.

Life will still be unpredictable, but it will have more flow, less resistance and tension. You'll have a new capacity to ease up on yourself. An average day will feel lighter, more hopeful, and more open-ended. Intuitive insight, understood in a practical way, will become as natural as breathing. You'll become a self-empowered being capable of fully participating in a co-creative process with life, as spirit merges with your humanness.

In the new days, once a critical mass of people have made a shift into heart awareness, life will be quite different for everyone. All of these benefits—and many more—are earned through systematically learning to focus on, listen to, and follow your heart.

# Glossary

**Amygdala:** The key subcortical brain center that coordinates behavioral, neural, immunological, and hormonal responses to environmental threats. It also serves as the storehouse of emotional memory within the brain. Its function is to compare incoming signals from the environment with stored emotional memories. In this way, the amygdala makes instantaneous decisions about the threat level of incoming sensory information. Due to its extensive connections to the hypothalamus and other autonomic nervous system centers, the amygdala is able to activate the autonomic nervous system and emotional responses before the higher brain centers receive the sensory information.

**Appreciation:** An active emotional state in which a person has clear perception or recognition of the quality or magnitude of that which he or she is thankful for. Appreciation also leads to improved physiological balance, as measured in cardiovascular and immune system function.

**Asset/Deficit Balance Sheet:** A HeartMath Solution tool for evaluating assets and deficits in relationship to how a person is using his or her mental and emotional energy. In conjunction with FREEZE-FRAME, the asset/deficit balance sheet can yield surprising insights and clarity on personal and professional issues.

**Atrial Natriuretic Factor (AND, or atrial peptide):** ANF, a hormone that regulates blood pressure, body fluid retention, and electrolyte homeostasis. It's nicknamed the "balance hormone." This hormone affects the blood vessels, the kidneys, the adrenal glands, and many regulatory areas in the brain.

**Autonomic Nervous System:** The portion of the nervous system that regulates most of the body's involuntary functions, including mean heart rate, the movements of the gastrointestinal tract, and the secretions of many glands. Consisting of two branches (the sympathetic and parasympathetic), the autonomic nervous system regulates over 90 percent of the body's functions. The heart and brain and the immune, hormonal, respiratory, and digestive systems are all connected by this network of nerves.

**Balance:** Stability, equilibrium, or the even distribution of weight on each side of a vertical axis. This term is also used to denote mental or emotional stability.

**Cardiac Coherence:** A mode of cardiac function in which the heart's rhythmic and electrical output is highly ordered. HeartMath research has shown that positive emotions such as love, care, and appreciation increase coherence in the heart's rhythmic beating patterns. During states of cardiac coherence, brain wave patterns have been shown to entrain with heart rate variability patterns; in addition, nervous system balance and immune function are enhanced. Overall, the body functions with increased harmony and efficiency.

**Cardiovascular System:** The system in the human body comprised of the heart and the blood vessels.

**Care:** an inner attitude or feeling of true service, without agendas or attachments to the outcome. Sincere care is rejuvenating for both the giver and recipient.

**Cell:** The smallest structural unit of an organism that's capable of independent functioning. The cell is a complex unit of protoplasm, usually having a nucleus, cytoplasm, and an enclosing membrane.

**Cellular:** Containing or consisting of cells.

**Cerebral Cortex:** The most highly developed area of the brain, governing all higher-order human capabilities, such as language, creativity, and problem-solving. The cortex, like other brain centers, continues to develop new neural circuits, or networks, throughout a person's life.

**Chaos:** Great disorder or confusion; incoherence. This term comes from the Greek word *khaos*, meaning "unformed matter." Chaos is the disordered state held to have existed before the ordered universe.

**Coherence:** Logical connectedness, internal order, or harmony among the components of a system. This term can also refer to the tendency toward increased order in the informational content of a system or in the information flow between systems. In physics, two or more wave forms that are phase-locked together (so that their energy is constructive) are described as coherent. Coherence can also be attributed to a single wave form, in which case it denotes an ordered or constructive distribution of power content. Recently, there has been a growing scientific interest in coherence in living systems. When a system is coherent, virtually no energy is wasted, because of the internal synchronization among the parts. In organizations, increased coherence enables the emergence of new levels of creativity, cooperation, productivity, and quality at all levels.

**Core Heart Feelings:** Psychological qualities commonly associated with the heart. These qualities represent some of the most beneficial and productive human values and traits. There are many core heart feelings, including love, compassion, nonjudgment, courage, patience, forgiveness, appreciation, and care.

**Cortical Inhibition:** Desynchronization or reduction of cortical activity, believed to result from the erratic heart rhythms and resulting neural signals transmitted from the heart to the brain during stress and negative emotional states. This condition can manifest in less efficient decision-making capabilities, leading to poor or short-sighted decisions, ineffective or impulsive communication, and reduced physical coordination.

**Cortisol:** A hormone produced by the adrenal glands during stressful situations, commonly known as the "stress hormone." Excessive cortisol has many harmful effects on the body and can destroy brain cells in the hippocampus, a region of the brain associated with learning and memory.

**DHEA:** An essential hormone produced by the adrenal glands and known as the "vitality hormone" because of its anti-aging properties. As the body's natural antagonist of the glucocorticoid hormones—a family that includes cortisol—DHEA reverses many of the unfavorable physiological effects of excessive stress. It's the precursor of the sex hormones estrogen and testosterone, and its varied functions include stimulation of the immune system, lowering of cholesterol levels, and promotion of bone and muscle deposition. Low DHEA levels have been reported in patients with many major diseases.

DNA: A complex molecule found in every cell of the body, carrying the genetic information or blueprint determining individual hereditary characteristics. An essential component of all living matter (and the major constituent of chromosomes), DNA is a nucleic acid consisting of two long chains of nucleotides twisted into a double helix.

Electromagnetic Signal: In physics, a wave propagated through space or matter by the oscillating electric and magnetic field generated by an oscillating electrical charge. In the human body, the heart is the most powerful source of electromagnetic energy.

Emotion: A strong feeling. Emotions include any of various complex reactions with both mental and physical manifestations—examples include love, joy, sorrow, and anger. Emotional energy is neutral, attaching itself to positive or negative thoughts to create *emotions*.

Emotional Management: The degree of ability one has to consciously control emotional responses.

Entrainment: A phenomenon seen throughout nature, whereby systems or organisms exhibiting periodic behavior come into sync, oscillating at the same frequency and phase. A common example of this phenomenon is the synchronization of two or more pendulum clocks placed near each other. In human beings, the entrainment of different oscillating biological systems to the primary frequency of the heart rhythms is often observed during positive emotional states. Entrainment, a highly efficient mode of bodily function, is associated with heightened clarity, buoyancy, and inner peace. Entrained teams are those that operate with a higher degree of synchronization, efficiency, and coherent communication.

FREEZE-FRAME: A key tool that consists of consciously disengaging one's mental and emotional reactions to either external or internal events and then shifting the center of attention from the mind and emotions to the physical area around the heart while focusing on a positive emotion such as love or appreciation. This tool is designed to prevent and release stress (by stopping nonefficient reactions in the moment) and then provide a window of opportunity for new, intuitive perspectives. FREEZE-FRAME has numerous applications for creative thinking, innovation, and planning, as well as improving overall health and well-being.

Frequency: The number of times any action, occurrence, or event is repeated in a given period. In physics, frequency is the number of periodic oscillations, vibrations, or waves per unit of time, usually expressed in cycles per second. Human intelligence operates within a large bandwidth of frequencies.

Head: Generally used to describe the brain and mind—that part of our intelligence that operates in a linear, logical manner. The head's primary functions are to analyze, memorize, compartmentalize, compare, and sort incoming messages from our senses and past experiences, which it then transforms into perceptions, thoughts, and emotions.

Heart: A hollow, muscular organ in vertebrates that keeps the blood in circulation throughout the body by means of its rhythmic contractions and relaxations. The body's central and most powerful energy generator and rhythmic oscillator, the heart is a complex, self-organized information-processing system with its own functional "little brain" that continually transmits neural, hormonal, rhythmic, and pressure messages to the brain.

**Heart/Brain Entrainment:** A state in which very low frequency brain waves and heart rhythms are frequency-locked—that is, entrained. This phenomenon has been associated with significant shifts in perception and heightened intuitive awareness.

**Heart Intelligence:** A term coined to express the concept of the heart as an intelligent system with the power to bring both the emotional and the mental systems into balance and coherence.

**HEART LOCK-IN:** A key technique used for quieting the mind and sustaining a solid connection with the heart, *locking in* to the heart's power. HEART LOCK-IN adds buoyancy and regenerative energy to a person's entire system.

**Heart Power Tools:** Core heart feelings that can be applied to activate heart intelligence, eliminate energy deficits, and increase energy assets.

**Heart Rate Variability (HRV):** The normally occurring beat-to-beat changes in heart rate. Analysis of HRV is an important tool used to assess the function and balance of the autonomic nervous system. HRV is considered a key indicator of aging, cardiac health, and overall well-being.

**Hormonal System:** Made up of the many hormones that act and interact throughout the body to regulate many metabolic functions, and the cells, organs, and tissues that manufacture them. (A hormone is a substance produced by living cells that circulates in the body fluids and produces a specific effect on the activity of cells remote from its point of origin.)

**Immune System:** The integrated bodily system of organs, tissues, cells, and cell products, such as antibodies, that differentiates "self" from "nonself" within our body and neutralizes potentially pathogenic organisms or substances that cause disease. The organizational "immune system" is built upon the core values known to enhance personal fulfillment and well-being, eliminating the emotional viruses that can permeate and destroy the effectiveness and coherence of the organization.

**Insight:** The faculty of seeing into inner character or underlying truth and apprehending the true nature of a thing. A clear understanding or awareness.

**Internal Coherence:** A deep state of internal self-management in which one generates increased order and harmony in the physical, mental, and emotional systems. In this state, the cardiovascular, immune, hormonal, and nervous systems function with heightened efficiency. States of internal coherence are associated with reduced emotional reactivity and greater mental clarity, creativity, adaptability, and flexibility.

**Internal Self-Management:** The active process of reducing and neutralizing one's automatic mental and emotional reactions to events or situations, instead of falling victim to them.

**Intuition:** Intelligence and understanding that bypasses the logical, linear cognitive processes; the faculty of direct knowing, as if by instinct, without conscious reasoning. Intuition is pure, untaught, inferential knowledge married to keen and quick insight.

**Intuitive Intelligence:** A type of intelligence distinct from cognitive processes, which derives from the consistent use and application of one's intuition. Research is showing that the human capacity to meet life's challenges with fluidity and grace is based not on knowledge, logic, or reason alone; it also includes the ability to make intuitive decisions. HeartMath research suggests that with training and practice, human beings can develop a high level of operational intuitive intelligence.

**Judgments:** Strongly held, largely negative attitudes and opinions often based on incomplete and prejudicial information.

**Limbic System:** A group of cortical and subcortical brain structures involved in emotional processing and certain aspects of memory. These structures include the hypothalamus, thalamus, hippocampus, and amygdala, among others.

**Nervous System:** The system of cells, tissues, and organs that coordinates and regulates the body's responses to internal and external stimuli. In vertebrates, the nervous system is made up of the brain and spinal cord, nerves, ganglia, and nerve centers in receptor and effector organs.

**Neural Circuits:** Neural pathways consisting of interconnected neurons in the brain and body through which specific information is processed. Research has shown that many of these neural connections develop in early childhood based on our experiences and the type of stimulation we receive. Likewise, even later in life, neural circuits can either be reinforced or atrophy, depending on how frequently we use them. Specific circuits form and are reinforced through repeated behavior, and in this way both physical and emotional responses can become "hardwired" (or automatic) in our system.

**Neuron:** Any of the cells that make up the nervous system, consisting of a nucleated cell body with one or more dendrites and a single axon. Neurons are the fundamental structural and functional units of nervous tissue.

**Neutral:** In physics, having a net electric charge of zero; with reference to machinery, a position in which a set of gears is disengaged. In human beings, going to a neutral state means consciously disengaging from our automatic mental and emotional reactions to a situation or issue in order to gain a wider perspective.

**Organizational Incoherence:** A state resulting from accumulated internal noise, turmoil, pressure, and conflict among the individuals that comprise the organization. This state is characterized by distorted perception, high levels of emotional reactivity, and decreased efficiency, cooperation, and productivity.

**Overcare:** The result of care taken to an inefficient extreme that crosses the line into anxiety and worry. Overcare is one of the greatest inhibitors of personal and organizational resilience. It's become so natural that people often don't know they're experiencing it, because it presents itself as care. As individuals learn to identify and plug the leaks in their own personal system caused by overcare, they stop draining energy and effectiveness, personally and organizationally.

**Parasympathetic:** The branch of the autonomic nervous system that slows or relaxes bodily functions. This part of the nervous system is analogous to the brakes in a car. Many known diseases and disorders are associated with diminished parasympathetic function.

**Perception:** The act or faculty of apprehending by means of the senses; the way in which an individual views a situation or event. How we perceive an event or an issue underlies how we think, feel, and react to that event or issue. Our level of awareness determines both our initial perception of an event and our ability to extract meaning from the available data. Research is showing that when the mind's logic and intellect are harmoniously integrated with the heart's intuitive intelligence, our perception of situations often changes significantly, offering wider perspectives and new possibilities.

**Quantum Theory:** A mathematical theory that describes the behavior of physical systems and is particularly useful in studying the energetic characteristics of matter at the subatomic level. One of the key principles of quantum theory is that we're not merely *observing* reality but are *participating* in the way we *create* our reality.

**Solar Plexus:** The large network of nerves located in the area of the belly just below the sternum; named due to the raylike patterns of its nerve fibers. This neural network is distributed throughout the tissue lining the esophagus, stomach, small intestine, and colon and is sometimes called the "enteric nervous system" or the "gut-brain."

**Stress:** Pressure, strain, or a sense of inner turmoil resulting from our perceptions and reactions to events or conditions. A state of negative emotional arousal, usually associated with feelings of discomfort or anxiety that we attribute to our circumstances or situation.

**Sympathetic:** The branch of the autonomic nervous system that speeds up the bodily functions, preparing us for mobilization and action. The fight-or-flight response to stress activates the sympathetic nervous system and causes the contraction of blood vessels, along with a rise in heart rate and many other bodily responses. This part of the nervous system is analogous to the gas pedal in a car.

**Time Shift:** Used here to describe the time saved when we're able to disengage from an inefficient mental or emotional reaction and make a more efficient choice. Time-shifting stops a chain-link reaction of time and energy waste and catapults people into a new domain of time management, where there's greater energy efficiency and fulfillment.

# References

## Chapter 1: Beyond the Brain—The Intelligent Heart

1. Dossey, L. *Space, Time & Medicine*. Boston: Shambhala, 1985; p. 11.

2. Saint-Exupéry, A. de. *The Little Prince*. San Diego: Harcourt Brace Jovanovich, 1943; quote p. 70.

2a. Carr, S., The Heart as Monarch, The Prime Meridian, Winter 1996; p. 1-13.

3. Schiefelbein, S. The powerful river. In: Poole, R., ed. *The Incredible Machine*. Washington, D.C.: The National Geographic Society, 1986.

4. Armour, J., and Ardell, J., eds. *Neurocardiology*. New York: Oxford University Press, 1984.

5. LeDoux, J. *The Emotional Brain: The Mysterious Underpinnings of Emotional Life*. New York: Simon & Schuster, 1996.

6. Lacey, J., and Lacey, B. Some autonomic–central nervous system interrelationships. In: Black, P., *Physiological Correlates of Emotion*. New York: Academic Press, 1970:205–227.

7. Frysinger, R. C., and Harper, R. M. Cardiac and respiratory correlations with unit discharge in epileptic human temporal lobe. *Epilepsia*. 1990;31(2):162–171.

8. Schandry, R., Sparrer, B., and Weitkunat, R. From the heart to the brain: a study of heartbeat contingent scalp potentials. *International Journal of Neuroscience*. 1986;30:261–275.

9. McCraty, R., Tiller, W. A., and Atkinson, M. Head-heart entrainment: A preliminary survey. In: *Proceedings of the Brain-Mind Applied Neurophysiology EEG Neurofeedback Meeting*. Key West, FL, 1996.

10. Rosenfeld, S. A. *Conversations Between Heart and Brain*. Rockville, MD: National Institute of Mental Health, 1977; quote p. ii.

11. Goleman, D. *Emotional Intelligence*. NY: Bantam Books, 1995; quote p. 47.

12. Gardner, H. *Frames of Mind*. New York: Basic Books, 1985.

13. Mayer, J., and Salovey, P. Emotional intelligence. *Applied and Preventive Psychology*. 1995;4(3):197–208.

14. Bar-On, R. The era of the "EQ": Defining and assessing emotional intelligence. Presented at the 104th Annual Convention of the American Psychological Association, Toronto, 1996.

15. McCraty, R., Atkinson, M., Tiller, W. A., and others. The effects of emotions on short-term heart rate variability using power spectrum analysis. *American Journal of Cardiology*. 1995;76:1089–1093.

16. McCraty, R., Atkinson, M., and Tiller, W. A. New electrophysiological correlates associated with intentional heart focus. *Subtle Energies*. 1995;4(3):251–268.

17. Tiller, W., McCraty, R., and Atkinson, M. Cardiac coherence: A new non-invasive measure of autonomic system order. *Alternative Therapies in Health and Medicine*. 1996; 2(1):52–65.

18. McCraty, R., Barrios-Choplin, B., Rozman, D., and others. The impact of a new emotional self-management program on stress, emotions, heart rate variability, DHEA, and cortisol. *Integrative Physiological and Behavioral Science*. 1998;33(2):151–170.

19. Rein, G., Atkinson, M., and McCraty, R. The physiological and psychological effects of compassion and anger. *Journal of Advancement in Medicine*. 1995;8(2):87–105.

20. Medalie, J. H., and Goldbourt, U. Angina pectoris among 10,000 men. II. Psychosocial and other risk factors as evidenced by a multivariate analysis of a five-year incidence study. *American Journal of Medicine*. 1976;60(6):910–921.

21. Medalie, J. H., Stange, K. C., Zyzanski, S. J., and others. The importance of biopsychosocial factors in the development of duodenal ulcer in a cohort of middle-aged men. *American Journal of Epidemiology*. 1992;136(10):1280–1287.

22. House, J. S., Robbins, C., and Metzner, H. L. The association of social relationships and activities with mortality: prospective evidence from the Tecumseh Community Health Study. *American Journal of Epidemiology*. 1982;116(1):123–140.

23. Russek, L., and Schwartz, G. E. Perceptions of parental love and caring predict health status in midlife: A 35-year follow-up of the Harvard mastery of stress study. *Psychosomatic Medicine*. 1997;59(2):144–149.

24. Ornish, D. *Love and Survival: The Scientific Basis for the Healing Power of Intimacy.* New York: HarperCollins, 1998.

25. Barrios-Choplin, B., McCraty, R., and Cryer, B. A new approach to reducing stress and improving physical and emotional well being at work. *Stress Medicine*. 1997;13:193–201.

26. McCraty, R., and Watkins, A. *Autonomic Assessment Report Interpretation Guide.* Boulder Creek, CA: Institute of HeartMath,1996.

27. McCraty, R., Rozman, D., and Childre, D., eds. *HeartMath: A New Biobehavioral Intervention for Increasing Health and Personal Effectiveness—Increasing Coherence in the Human System* (working title). Amsterdam: Harwood Academic Publishers, 1999 (fall release).

## Chapter 2: The Ultimate Partnership

1. LeDoux, J. *The Emotional Brain: The Mysterious Underpinnings of Emotional Life.* New York: Simon & Schuster, 1996.

2. Atkinson, M. *Personal and Organizational Quality Survey Progress Report for CalPERS.* Boulder Creek, CA: HeartMath Research Center, 1998.

3. McCraty, R., Rozman, D., and Childre, D., eds. *HeartMath: A New Biobehavioral Intervention for Increasing Health and Personal Effectiveness—Increasing Coherence in the Human System* (working title). Amsterdam: Harwood Academic Publishers, 1999 (fall release).

4. Armour, J., and Ardell, J., eds. *Neurocardiology.* Oxford University Press: New York, 1994.

5. Armour, J. Anatomy and function of the intrathoracic neurons regulating the mammalian heart. In: Zucker, I., and Gilmore, J., eds. *Reflex Control of the Circulation.* Boca Raton, FL: CRC Press, 1991:1–37.

6. Armour, J. Neurocardiology: Anatomical and functional principles. In: McCraty, R., Rozman, D., and Childre, D., eds. *HeartMath: A New Biobehavioral Intervention for Increasing Health and Personal Effectiveness—Increasing Coherence in the Human System* (working title). Amsterdam: Harwood Academic Publishers, 1999 (fall release).

7. Lacey, J., and Lacey, B. Some autonomic–central nervous system interrelationships. In: Black, P., ed. *Physiological Correlates of Emotion.* New York: Academic Press, 1970:205–227.

8. Koriath, J., and Lindholm, E. Cardiac-related cortical inhibition during a fixed foreperiod reaction time task. *International Journal of Psychophysiology.* 1986;4:183–195.

9. Schandry, R., and Montoya, P. Event-related brain potentials and the processing of cardiac activity. *Biological Psychology.* 1996;42:75–85.

10. Frysinger, R. C., and Harper, R. M. Cardiac and respiratory correlations with unit discharge in epileptic human temporal lobe. *Epilepsia.* 1990;31(2):162–171.

11. Turpin, G. Cardiac-respiratory integration: Implications for the analysis and interpretation of phasic cardiac responses. In: Grossman, P., Janssen, K., and Vaitl, D., eds. *Cardiorespiratory and cardiosomatic psychophysiology.* New York: Plenum Press, 1985:139–155.

12. Cantin, M., and Genest, J. The heart as an endocrine gland. *Scientific American.* 1986;254(2):76–81.

13. Kellner, M., Wiedemann, K., and Holsboer, F. Atrial natriuretic factor inhibits the CRH-stimulated secretion of ACTH and cortisol in man. *Life Sciences.* 1992;50(24):1835–1842.

14. Kentsch, M., Lawrenz, R., Ball, P., and others. Effects of atrial natriuretic factor on anterior pituitary hormone secretion in normal man. *Clinical Investigator.* 1992;70:549–555.

15. Vollmar, A., Lang, R., Hänze, J., and others. A possible linkage of atrial natriuretic peptide to the immune system. *American Journal of Hypertension.* 1990;3(5 pt. 1):408–411.

16. Telegdy, G. The action of ANP, BNP, and related peptides on motivated behavior in rats. *Reviews in the Neurosciences.* 1994;5(4):309–315.

17. Huang, M., Friend, D., Sunday, M., and others. Identification of novel catecholamine-containing cells not associated with sympathetic neurons in cardiac muscle. *Circulation.* 1995;92(8):1–59.

18. Pert, C. *Molecules of Emotion.* New York: Scribner, 1997.

19. Langhorst, P., Schulz, G., and Lambertz, M. Oscillating neuronal network of the "common brainstem system." In: Miyakawa, K., Koepchen, H., and Polosa, C., eds. *Mechanisms of Blood Pressure Waves.* Tokyo: Japan Scientific Societies Press, 1984:257–275.

20. Song, L., Schwartz, G., and Russek, L. Heart-focused attention and heart-brain synchronization: Energetic and physiological mechanisms. *Alternative Therapies in Health and Medicine.* 1998;4(5):44–62.

21. McCraty, R., Tiller, W. A., and Atkinson, M. Head-heart entrainment: A preliminary survey. In: *Proceedings of the Brain-Mind Applied Neurophysiology EEG Neurofeedback Meeting.* Key West, FL, 1996.

22. McCraty, R., Atkinson, M., Tomasino, D., and others. The electricity of touch: Detection and measurement of cardiac energy exchange between people. In: Pribram, K., ed. *Brain and Values: Is a Biological Science of Values Possible?* Mahwah, NJ: Lawrence Erlbaum Associates, 1998:359–379.

23. Dekker, J. M., Schouten, E. G., Klootwijk, P., and others. Heart rate variability from short electrocardiographic recordings predicts mortality from all causes in middle-aged and elderly men. The Zutphen Study. *American Journal of Epidemiology.* 1997;145(10):899–908.

24. Umetani, K., Singer, D. H., McCraty, R., and others. Twenty-four-hour time domain heart rate variability and heart rate: Relations to age and gender over nine decades. *Journal of the American College of Cardiology.* 1998;31(3):593–601.

25. McCraty, R., Atkinson, M., Tiller, W. A., and others. The effects of emotions on short-term heart rate variability using power spectrum analysis. *American Journal of Cardiology.* 1995;76:1089–1093.

26. Tiller, W., McCraty, R., and Atkinson, M. Cardiac coherence: A new, noninvasive measure of autonomic nervous system order. *Alternative Therapies in Health and Medicine.* 1996;2(1):52–65.

27. American Heart Association. *1998 Heart and Stroke Statistical Update*. Dallas, TX: American Heart Association, 1997.

28. Rein, G., Atkinson, M., and McCraty, R. The physiological and psychological effects of compassion and anger. *Journal of Advancement in Medicine*. 1995;8(2):87–105.

29. McCraty, R., Atkinson, M., Rein, G., and others. Music enhances the effect of positive emotional states on salivary IgA. *Stress Medicine*. 1996;12:167–175.

30. McCraty, R., Barrios-Choplin, B., Rozman, D., and others. The impact of a new emotional self-management program on stress, emotions, heart rate variability, DHEA, and cortisol. *Integrative Physiological and Behavioral Science*. 1998;33(2):151–170.

31. Strogatz, S. H., and Stewart, I. Coupled oscillators and biological synchronization. *Scientific American*. 1993;269(6):102–109.

32. George, quoted in: Marquis, J. Our emotions: Why we feel the way we do; New advances are opening our subjective inner worlds to objective study. Discoveries are upsetting longheld notions. *Los Angeles Times*, Oct. 14, 1996, home ed., p. A-1.

## Chapter 3: The Risks of Incoherence

1. Childre, D., and Cryer, B. *From Chaos to Coherence: Advancing Emotional and Organizational Intelligence Through Inner Quality Management*. Boston: Butterworth-Heinnemann, 1998.

2. McCraty, R., Tiller, W. A., and Atkinson, M. Head-heart entrainment: A preliminary survey. In: *Proceedings of the Brain-Mind Applied Neurophysiology EEG Neurofeedback Meeting*. Key West, FL, 1996.

3. Cooper, C. *Handbook of Stress, Medicine, and Health*. Boca Raton, FL: CRC Press, 1996.

4. Hafen, B., Frandsen, K., Karren, K., and others. *The Health Effects of Attitudes, Emotions, and Relationships*. Provo, UT: EMS Associates, 1992.

5. Sterling, P., and Eyer, J. Biological basis of stress-related mortality. *Social Science and Medicine*. 1981;15E:3–42.

6. Rosch, P. Job stress: America's leading adult health problem. *USA Today*, May 1991, pp. 42–44.

7. Wayne, D. Reactions to stress. In: *Identifying Stress*, a series offered by the Health-Net & Stress Management Web site, Feb. 1998.

8. Rosenman, R. The independent roles of diet and serum lipids in the 20th-century rise and decline of coronary heart disease mortality. *Integrative Physiological and Behavioral Science*. 1993;28(1):84–98.

9. Eysenck, H. J. Personality, stress, and cancer: prediction and prophylaxis. *British Journal of Medical Psychology*. 1988;61(Pt 1):57–75.

10. Mittleman, M. A., Maclure, M., Sherwood, J. B., and others. Triggering of acute myocardial infarction onset by episodes of anger. *Circulation*. 1995;92(7):1720–1725.

11. Kubzansky, L. D., Kawachi, I., Spiro, A., III, and others. Is worrying bad for your heart? A prospective study of worry and coronary heart disease in the Normative Aging Study. *Circulation*. 1997;95(4):818–824.

12. Dixon, J., Dixon, J., and Spinner, J. Tensions between career and interpersonal commitments as a risk factor for cardiovascular disease among women. *Women and Health*. 1991;17:33–57.

13. Penninx, B. W., van Tilburg, T., Kriegsman, D. M., and others. Effects of social support and personal coping resources on mortality in older age: "The Longitudinal Aging Study Amsterdam." *American Journal of Epidemiology*. 1997;146(6):510–519.

14. Allison, T. G., Williams, D. E., Miller, T. D., and others. Medical and economic costs of psychologic distress in patients with coronary artery disease. *Mayo Clinic Proceedings.* 1995;70(8):734–742.

15. Gullette, E., Blumenthal, J., Babyak, M., and others. Effects of mental stress on myocardial ischemia during daily life. *Journal of the American Medical Association.* 1997; 277:1521–1526.

16. Mittleman, M., and Maclure, M. Mental stress during daily life triggers myocardial ischemia [editorial; comment]. *Journal of the American Medical Association.* 1997;277: 1558–1559; quote p. 1558.

17. Hiemke, C. Circadian variations in antigen-specific proliferation of human T lymphocytes and correlation to cortisol production. *Psychoneuroendocrinology.* 1994;20:335–342.

18. DeFeo, P. Contribution of cortisol to glucose counterregulation in humans. *American Journal of Physiology.* 1989;257:E35-E42.

19. Manolagas, S. C. Adrenal steroids and the development of osteoporosis in the oophorectomized women. *Lancet.* 1979;2:597.

20. Berne, R. *Physiology* (3rd ed.). St. Louis: Mosby, 1993.

21. Marin, P. Cortisol secretion in relation to body fat distribution in obese premenopausal women. *Metabolism.* 1992;41:882–886.

22. Kerr, D. S., Campbell, L. W., Applegate, M. D., and others. Chronic stress-induced acceleration of electrophysiologic and morphometric biomarkers of hippocampal aging. *Society of Neuroscience.* 1991;11(5):1316–1317.

23. Sapolsky, R. *Stress, the Aging Brain, and the Mechanisms of Neuron Death.* Cambridge, MA: MIT Press, 1992.

24. Nixon, P., and King, J. Ischemic heart disease: Homeostasis and the heart. In: Watkins, A., *Mind-Body Medicine: A Clinician's Guide to Psychoneuroimmunology.* New York: Churchill Livingstone, 1997:41–73.

25. Temoshok, L., and Dreher, H. *The Type C Connection: The Behavioral Links to Cancer and Your Health.* New York: Random House, 1992.

26. Carroll, D., Smith, G., Willemsen, G., and others. Blood pressure reactions to the cold pressor test and the prediction of ischemic heart disease: Data from the Caerphilly Study. *Journal of Epidemiology and Community Health.* Sept. 1998:528.

27. Siegman, A. W., Townsend, S. T., Blumenthal, R. S., and others. Dimensions of anger and CHD in men and women: Self-ratings versus spouse ratings. *Journal of Behavioral Medicine.* 1998;21(4):315–336.

28. Vest, J., and Cohen, W. Road rage. *U.S. News & World Report,* May 25, 1997, pp. 24–30.

29. Pearsall, P. *The Heart's Code.* New York: Broadway Books, 1998.

30. Williams, R. *Anger Kills.* New York: Times Books, 1993.

31. Tiller, W., McCraty, R., and Atkinson, M. Cardiac coherence: A new non-invasive measure of autonomic system order. *Alternative Therapies in Health and Medicine.* 1996;2(1):52–65.

32. McCraty, R., Atkinson, M., and Tiller, W. A. New electrophysiological correlates associated with intentional heart focus. *Subtle Energies.* 1995;4(3):251–268.

33. Burrows, G. Stress in the professional. In: *Seventh International Congress on Stress.* Montreux, Switzerland: The American Institute of Stress, 1995.

## Chapter 4: FREEZE-FRAME

1. Thomson, B. Change of heart. *Natural Health,* Sept./Oct. 1997:98–103.

2. Childre, D. FREEZE-FRAME®: *A Scientifically Proven Technique for Clear Decision Making and Improved Health.* Boulder Creek, CA: Planetary Publications, 1998.

3. McCraty, R., Atkinson, M., Tiller, W. A., and others. The effects of emotions on short-term heart rate variability using power spectrum analysis. *American Journal of Cardiology.* 1995,76.1089–1093.

4. McCraty, R., Tiller, W. A., and Atkinson, M. Head-heart entrainment: A preliminary survey. In: *Proceedings of the Brain-Mind Applied Neurophysiology EEG Neurofeedback Meeting.* Key West, FL, 1996.

5. McCraty, R., Atkinson, M., and Tiller, W. A. New electrophysiological correlates associated with intentional heart focus. *Subtle Energies.* 1995;4(3):251–268.

6. Tiller, W., McCraty, R., and Atkinson, M. Cardiac coherence: A new non-invasive measure of autonomic system order. *Alternative Therapies in Health and Medicine.* 1996;2(1):52–65.

7. McCraty, R., Atkinson, M., Rein, G., and others. Music enhances the effect of positive emotional states on salivary IgA. *Stress Medicine.* 1996;12:167–175.

8. Rein, G., Atkinson, M., and McCraty, R. The physiological and psychological effects of compassion and anger. *Journal of Advancement in Medicine.* 1995;8(2):87–105.

9. Raschke, F. The hierarchical order of cardiovascular-respiratory coupling. In: Grossman, P., Janssen, K.H.L., and Vaitl, D., eds. *Cardiorespiratory and cardiosomatic psychophysiology.* New York: Plenum Press, 1985:207–217.

**Chapter 5: Energy Efficiency**

1. Sterling, P., and Eyer, J. Biological basis of stress-related mortality. *Social Science and Medicine.* 1981;15E:3–42.

2. Kiecolt-Glaser, J. K., Stephens, R. E., Lipetz, P. D., and others. Distress and DNA repair in human lymphocytes. *Journal of Behavioral Medicine.* 1985;8(4):311–320.

3. Sapolsky, R. *Stress, the Aging Brain, and the Mechanisms of Neuron Death.* Cambridge, MA: MIT Press, 1992.

4. Tiller, W., McCraty, R., and Atkinson, M. Cardiac coherence: A new non-invasive measure of autonomic system order. *Alternative Therapies in Health and Medicine.* 1996; 2(1):52–65.

5. Atkinson, M. *Personal and Organizational Quality Survey Progress Report for CalPERS.* Boulder Creek, CA: HeartMath Research Center, 1998.

6. Atkinson, M. *Personal and Organizational Quality Survey Progress Report for Department of Justice, Workers Compensation Study.* Boulder Creek, CA: HeartMath Research Center, 1997.

7. Atkinson, M. *Personal and Organizational Quality Survey Progress Report for Internal Revenue Service.* Boulder Creek, CA: HeartMath Research Center, 1997.

8. McCraty, R., Barrios-Choplin, B., Rozman, D., and others. The impact of a new emotional self-management program on stress, emotions, heart rate variability, DHEA, and cortisol. *Integrative Physiological and Behavioral Science.* 1998;33(2):151–170.

9. McCraty, R., Barrios-Choplin, B., Atkinson, M., and others. The effects of different types of music on mood, tension, and mental clarity. *Alternative Therapies in Health and Medicine.* 1998;4(1):75–84.

10. Kiecolt-Glaser, J. K., Malarkey, W. B., Chee, M., and others. Negative behavior during marital conflict is associated with immunological down-regulation. *Psychosomatic Medicine.* 1993;55(5):395–409.

11. Kiecolt-Glaser, J. K., Glaser, R., Cacioppo, J. T., and others. Marital stress: Immunologic, neuroendocrine, and autonomic correlates. *Annals of the New York Academy of Sciences*. 1998;840:656–663.

12. Malarkey, W. B., Kiecolt-Glaser, J. K., Pearl, D., and others. Hostile behavior during marital conflict alters pituitary and adrenal hormones. *Psychosomatic Medicine*. 1994;56(1): 41–51.

13. Rosenman, R. H., Brand, R. J., Jenkins, D., and others. Coronary heart disease in Western Collaborative Group Study. Final follow-up experience of 8 1/2 years. *JAMA*. 1975;233(8):872–877.

14. Barefoot, J. C., Dahlstrom, W. G., and Williams, R. B., Jr. Hostility, CHD incidence, and total mortality: a 25-year follow-up study of 255 physicians. *Psychosomatic Medicine*. 1983;45(1):59–63.

15. Rein, G., Atkinson, M., and McCraty, R. The physiological and psychological effects of compassion and anger. *Journal of Advancement in Medicine*. 1995;8(2):87–105.

## Chapter 6: At the Heart's Core: The Power Tools of the Heart

1. Cathcart, J. *The Acorn Principle*. New York: St. Martin's Press, 1998; quote p. 179.

## Chapter 7: Understanding the Mystery of Emotions

1. *Stedman's Medical Dictionary*, 25th ed. Baltimore: Williams & Wilkins, 1990.

2. LeDoux, J. E. Emotion, memory, and the brain. *Scientific American*. 1994;270(6): 50–57.

3. Benson, H. *Timeless Healing*. New York: Scribner, 1996.

4. *The Random House College Dictionary*. New York: Random House, 1995.

5. LeDoux, J. *The Emotional Brain: The Mysterious Underpinnings of Emotional Life*. New York: Simon & Schuster, 1996.

6. LeDoux, J. E. Emotional memory systems in the brain. *Behavioural Brain Research*. 1993;58(1–2):69–79.

7. Oppenheimer, S., and Hopkins, D. Suprabulbar neuronal regulation of the heart. In: Armour, J. A., and Ardell, J. L., eds. *Neurocardiology*. New York: Oxford University Press, 1994:309–341.

8. Pribram, K. H. *Brain and Perception: Holonomy and Structure in Figural Processing*. Hillsdale, NJ: Lawrence Erlbaum Associates, 1991.

9. Pert, C. *Molecules of Emotion*. New York: Scribner, 1997.

10. Frysinger, R. C., and Harper, R. M. Cardiac and respiratory correlations with unit discharge in epileptic human temporal lobe. *Epilepsia*. 1990;31(2):162–171.

11. McCraty, R., Barrios-Choplin, B., Rozman, D., and others. The impact of a new emotional self-management program on stress, emotions, heart rate variability, DHEA, and cortisol. *Integrative Physiological and Behavioral Science*. 1998;33(2):151–170.

12. McCraty, R., Atkinson, M., and Tiller, W. A. New electrophysiological correlates associated with intentional heart focus. *Subtle Energies*. 1995;4(3):251–268.

13. McCraty, R., Tiller, W. A., and Atkinson, M. Head-heart entrainment: A preliminary survey. In: *Proceedings of the Brain-Mind Applied Neurophysiology EEG Neurofeedback Meeting*. Key West, FL, 1996.

14. Tiller, W., McCraty, R., and Atkinson, M. Cardiac coherence: A new non-invasive measure of autonomic system order. *Alternative Therapies in Health and Medicine*. 1996; 2(1):52–65.

15. Lessmeier, T. J., Gamperling, D., Johnson-Liddon, V., and others. Unrecognized paroxysmal supraventricular tachycardia: potential for misdiagnosis as panic disorder. *Archives of Internal Medicine*. 1997;157:537–543.

16. Goleman, D. *Emotional Intelligence*. NY: Bantam Books, 1995.

## Chapter 8: Care Versus Overcare

1. McCraty, R., Atkinson, M., Tomasino, D., and others. The electricity of touch: Detection and measurement of cardiac energy exchange between people. In: Pribram, K., ed. *Brain and Values: Is a Biological Science of Values Possible?* Mahwah, NJ: Lawrence Erlbaum Associates, 1998:359–379.

2. McCraty, R., Rozman, D., and Childre, D., eds. *HeartMath: A New Biobehavioral Intervention for Increasing Health and Personal Effectiveness—Increasing Coherence in the Human System* (working title). Amsterdam: Harwood Academic Publishers, 1999 (fall release).

3. Russek, L., and Schwartz, G. Interpersonal heart-brain registration and the perception of parental love: A 42 year follow-up of the Harvard Mastery of Stress Study. *Subtle Energies*. 1994;5(3):195–208.

4. Tiller, W., McCraty, R., and Atkinson, M. Cardiac coherence: A new, noninvasive measure of autonomic nervous system order. *Alternative Therapies in Health and Medicine*. 1996;2(1):52–65.

5. Quinn, J. Building a body of knowledge: Research on Therapeutic Touch 1974–1986. *Journal of Holistic Nursing*. 1988;6(1):37–45.

6. The human touch researchers at the University of Miami have drawn nationwide attention for their studies showing the powerful benefits of massage for premature infants, full-term babies, and children. *(Ft. Lauderdale) Sun-Sentinel*, Jan. 18, 1998.

7. Field, T. Massage therapy for infants and children. *Journal of Developmental Behavioral Pediatrics*. 1995;16(2):105–111.

8. Ironson, G., Field, T., Scafidi, F., and others. Massage therapy is associated with enhancement of the immune system's cytotoxic capacity. *International Journal of Neuroscience*. 1996;84(1–4):205–217.

9. Field, T., Ironson, G., Scafidi F., and others. Massage therapy reduces anxiety and enhances EEG pattern of alertness and math computations. *International Journal of Neuroscience*. 1996;86(3–4):197–205.

10. Green, J., and Shellenberger, R. The subtle energy of love. *Subtle Energies*. 1993; 4(1):31–55.

11. Hafen, B., Frandsen, K., Karren, K., and others. *The Health Effects of Attitudes, Emotions, and Relationships*. Provo, UT: EMS Associates, 1992.

12. Ornish, D. *Love and Survival: The Scientific Basis for the Healing Power of Intimacy*. New York: HarperCollins, 1998.

13. Friedmann, E., and Thomas, S. A. Pet ownership, social support, and one-year survival after acute myocardial infarction in the Cardiac Arrhythmia Suppression Trial (CAST). *American Journal of Cardiology*. 1995;76(17):1213–1217.

14. Melson, G., Peet, S., and Sparks, C. Children's attachment to their pets: Links to socio-emotional development. *Children's Environments Quarterly*. 1991;8(2):55–65.

15. McClelland, D. C., and Kirshnit, C. The effects of motivational arousal through films on salivary immunoglobulin A. *Psychological Health*. 1988;2:31–52.

16. Rein, G., Atkinson, M., and McCraty, R. The physiological and psychological effects of compassion and anger. *Journal of Advancement in Medicine*. 1995;8(2):87–105.

## Chapter 9: CUT-THRU to Emotional Maturity

1. LeDoux, J. *The Emotional Brain: The Mysterious Underpinnings of Emotional Life.* New York: Simon & Schuster, 1996.

2. Blakeslee, S. Complex and hidden brain in the gut makes stomachaches and butterflies. *New York Times,* Jan. 23, 1996; quote p. C-3.

3. McCraty, R., Barrios-Choplin, B., Rozman, D., and others. The impact of a new emotional self-management program on stress, emotions, heart rate variability, DHEA, and cortisol. *Integrative Physiological and Behavioral Science.* 1998;33(2):151–170.

4. Ebbinghaus, H. *Memory. A Contribution to Experimental Psychology.* New York: Dover, 1963 (repr.), 1885.

5. Kandel, E. Genes, nerve cells, and the remembrance of things past. *Journal of Neuropsychiatry.* 1989;1(2):103–125.

6. Schacter, D. Memory and awareness. *Science.* 1998;280(3):59–60.

7. Pert, C. *Molecules of Emotion.* New York: Scribner, 1997.

8. Compound being tested could ease aches of aging. *San Jose (CA) Mercury News,* Sept. 3, 1995.

9. Shealy, N. A review of dehydroepiandrosterone (DHEA). *Integrative Physiological and Behavioral Science.* 1995;30(4):308–313.

10. Kerr, D. S., Campbell, L. W., Applegate, M. D., and others. Chronic stress-induced acceleration of electrophysiologic and morphometric biomarkers of hippocampal aging. *Society of Neuroscience.* 1991;11(5):1316–1317.

11. Marin, P. Cortisol secretion in relation to body fat distribution in obese premenopausal women. *Metabolism.* 1992;41:882–886.

12. Namiki, M. Biological markers of aging. *Nippon Ronen Igakkai Zasshi.* 1994;31:85–95.

13. Childre, D. L. *Speed of Balance: A Musical Adventure for Emotional and Mental Regeneration.* Boulder Creek, CA: Planetary Publications, 1995.

14. Childre, D. L. *CUT-THRU.* Boulder Creek, CA: Planetary Publications, 1996.

## Chapter 10: HEART LOCK-IN

1. Paddison, S. *The Hidden Power of the Heart.* Boulder Creek, CA: Planetary Publications, 1992.

2. Kauffman, D. Face to face: Interview with Everett Koop. *Science & Spirit.* 1997; 9(3):9.

3. Ornish, D. *Love and Survival: The Scientific Basis for the Healing Power of Intimacy.* New York: HarperCollins, 1998.

4. Myers, D., Psychology, applied spirituality, and health: Do they relate? *Science & Spirit.* 1998;9(3):30.

5. Benson, H. *Timeless Healing.* New York: Scribner, 1996.

6. Dossey, L. *Healing Words.* San Francisco: HarperCollins, 1993; quote p. 97.

7. McCraty, R., Atkinson, M., Rein, G., and others. Music enhances the effect of positive emotional states on salivary IgA. *Stress Medicine.* 1996;12:167–175.

8. McCraty, R., Barrios-Choplin, B., Atkinson, M., and others. The effects of different types of music on mood, tension, and mental clarity. *Alternative Therapies in Health and Medicine.* 1998;4(1):75–84.

9. McCraty, R., Barrios-Choplin, B., Rozman, D., and others. The impact of a new emotional self-management program on stress, emotions, heart rate variability, DHEA, and cortisol. *Integrative Physiological and Behavioral Science.* 1998;33(2):151–170.

10. Tomasi, T. *The Immune System of Secretions*. New Jersey: Prentice-Hall, 1976.

11. Childre, D. L. *Heart Zones*. Boulder Creek, CA: Planetary Publications, 1991.

## Chapter 11: Families, Children, and the Heart

1. Childre, D. L. *A Parenting Manual*. Boulder Creek, CA: Planetary Publications, 1995.

2. *National Survey on Communicating Family Values*, sponsored by Massachusetts Mutual Insurance Company, Dec. 1992; quote p. 4.

3. Balancing work and family. *Business Week*, Sept. 16, 1996.

4. Sacks, M. Sensory overload: Many hours in the fast lane render '90s kids bored, restless. *San Jose (CA) Mercury News*, Mar. 10, 1998.

5. Resnick, M. D., Bearman, P. S., Blum, R. W., and others. Protecting adolescents from harm. Findings from the National Longitudinal Study on Adolescent Health. *Journal of the American Medical Association*. 1997;278(10):823–832.

6. Russek, L., and Schwartz, G. E. Perceptions of parental love and caring predict health status in midlife: A 35-year follow-up of the Harvard mastery of stress study. *Psychosomatic Medicine*. 1997;59(2):144–149.

7. Brownlee, S. Invincible kids. *U.S. News & World Report*, Nov. 11, 1996.

8. Beidel, D. C., and Turner, S. M. At risk for anxiety: I. Psychopathology in the offspring of anxious parents. *Journal of the American Academy of Child and Adolescent Psychiatry*. 1997;36(7):918–924.

9. Childre, D. *Teaching Children to Love*. Boulder Creek, CA: Planetary Publications, 1996.

## Chapter 12: Social Impact

1. Taking the stress out of being stressed out. *Business Week Health Wire*, Mar. 20, 1997.

2. Rucci, A. J., Kirn, S. P., and Quinn, R. T. The employee-customer-profit chain at Sears. *Harvard Business Review*. 1998;Jan/Feb:82.

3. Childre, D., and Cryer, B. *From Chaos to Coherence: Advancing Emotional and Organizational Intelligence Through Inner Quality Management*. Boston: Butterworth-Heinnemann, 1998; quote p. 4.

4. Barrios-Choplin, B., McCraty, R., and Cryer, B. A new approach to reducing stress and improving physical and emotional well being at work. *Stress Medicine*. 1997;13:193–201.

5. Arnsten, A. The biology of being frazzled. *Science*. 1998;280(5370):1711–1712.

## Chapter 13: The 21st-Century Heart

1. Bohm, D., and Hiley, B. J. *The Undivided Universe*. London: Routledge, 1993; quote p. 382.

2. McCraty, R., Rozman, D., and Childre, D., eds. *HeartMath: A New Biobehavioral Intervention for Increasing Health and Personal Effectiveness—Increasing Coherence in the Human System* (working title). Amsterdam: Harwood Academic Publishers, 1999 (fall release).

3. Sheldrake, R. *A New Science of Life*. Los Angeles: Tarcher, 1981.

4. Penrose, R. *Shadows of the Mind: A Search for the Missing Science of Consciousness*. Oxford: Oxford University Press, 1994.

5. Hameroff, S. R. "More neural than thou": Reply to Patricia Churland's "Brainshy." In: Hameroff, S., Kaszniak, A., and Scott, A. C., eds. *Toward a Science of Consciousness II*. Cambridge, MA: MIT Press, 1998.

6. Gough, W. C., and Shacklett, R. L. The science of connectiveness; Part III: the human experience. *Subtle Energies*. 1993;4(3):187–214.

7. Tiller, W. A. *Science and Human Transformation*. Walnut Creek, CA: Pavior Publishing, 1997.

# Learning More About
# the HeartMath Experience

**Log on to http://www.heartmathsolution.com
and find out about HeartMath events in your area,
communicate with the authors, or learn more
about the HeartMath experience.**

### Retreats, Seminars, and Training Programs

HeartMath training programs are specifically designed to provide tools and techniques that increase productivity through enhanced job satisfaction, increased goal clarity, and improved health. The tools and techniques—designed for practical use in situations characterized by information overload, time pressure, and stress—reduce tension, fight burnout, and ameliorate physical symptoms of stress and negative moods.

HeartMath provides retreats, seminars, and off-site programs to help individuals and organizations discover and sustain the use of the HeartMath Solution. Inner Quality Management (IQM), the flagship organizational program, has a modular design that can be customized to fit an organization's specific business objectives.

For more information on trainings and seminars, call 1-800-450-9111 or write to:

HeartMath
14700 West Park Avenue
Boulder Creek, CA 95006
You can also visit our Web site: *http://www.heartmath.com*

### Books, Tapes, and Learning Programs

The HeartMath Solution, developed by Doc Childre, provides simple, proven tools and techniques to help people manage mental and emotional responses to life through the natural, commonsense intelligence of their own hearts. Explore and experience more of the HeartMath Solution with books, music, audiotapes, and learning programs.

HeartMath products can be used by individuals, small groups, or organizations to learn and sustain the skills necessary to function at a higher level of personal and organizational quality.

For a free catalog of our complete HeartMath product line or for information on volume discounts, call 1-800-372-3100 or write to:

Planetary Publications
P.O. Box 66
Boulder Creek, CA 95006

You can also visit our Web site *(http://www.planetarypub.com)* or reach us on-line at *info@planetarypub.com.*

Other books by Doc Childre:

*From Chaos to Coherence: Advancing Emotional and Organizational Intelligence through Inner Quality Management*
*Freeze-Frame: One Minute Stress Management*
*Teaching Children to Love: 80 Games & Fun Activities for Raising Balanced Children in Unbalanced Times*
*A Parenting Manual: Heart Hope for the Family*
*Teen Self Discovery: Helping Teens Find Balance, Security & Esteem*
*Self Empowerment: The Heart Approach to Stress Management*
*HeartMath Discovery Program: Daily Readings and Self-Discovery Exercises for Creating a More Rewarding Life*

## Support the HeartMath Experience

The Institute of HeartMath (IHM) is a nonprofit research organization that's revolutionizing our understanding of human intelligence and the role of the heart. Scientific studies conducted by IHM showing how the heart affects perception, information processing, and hormonal and immune system balance have been published in major medical journals, including *American Journal of Cardiology, Stress Medicine,* and *Journal of Advancement in Medicine.*

In addition, IHM is constructing a wellness clinic, conducts capital campaigns to support its research, and administers the HeartMath Hub program—a network of small study groups for developing heart intelligence.

The Institute of HeartMath has information on the following:

- Participating in or starting a Hub group in your area
- Contributing to a capital campaign
- Learning about IHM research and case studies
- Participating in volunteer programs

If you're interested in receiving information in one of these areas, call 831-338-8500, email us at *info@heartmath.org,* or write to:

Institute of HeartMath
P.O. Box 1463
Boulder Creek, CA 95006
You can also visit our Web site: *http://www.heartmath.org*